Healthy Choices, Healthy Schools

The Residential Curriculum

Edited by
Louis M. Crosier

1992
AVOCUS PUBLISHING, INC.
WASHINGTON, D.C.

HEALTHY CHOICES, HEALTHY SCHOOLS:
THE RESIDENTIAL CURRICULUM

Published by:

Avocus Publishing, Inc.
1223 Potomac Street, N.W.
Washington, D.C. 20007 USA
Telephone: 202-333-8190
Fax: 202-337-3809
Orders: 800-345-6665

Disclaimer:

Nothing contained in this book is intended in any way to be libelous in nature. Neither is it the intent of Avocus Publishing, Inc. to publish any accusatory statement, direct or implied, of improper motives or illegal actions by any individual or educational institution. Any other interpretation of our printing is erroneous and therefore misunderstood. We believe that the public interest in general and education in particular will be better served by the publication of the authors' experiences and analyses. Names of individuals other than the authors have been changed or omitted.

Copyright © 1992 by Avocus Publishing, Inc.
Printed in the United States of America

Library of Congress Catalog Card Number: 92-072463

ISBN 0-9627671-1-5: $19.95 Softcover

Cover design by Sharon Oleksiak

For Claire
Who turns problems into challenges,
disappointment into opportunity,
who loves exploring and finds joy in the simple things
that others pass by unknowing

For Chuck Kinyon
Who has taught me to thrive in the face of adversity

For Rich and Ginny Maxson
Who achieve excellence through honesty,
accountability and staff development and
who strive for truth in their work with children

For Ted Mitchell
Who cuts through rhetoric, bureaucracy and
facade to create solution-oriented schools

For John Rassias
Who colors outside the lines and
brings learning to life better than any teacher
I've ever had the opportunity to love

Acknowledgements

Producing *Healthy Choices, Healthy Schools* was a speedy project by normal publishing standards. Quick work requires considerable help and a coordinated team effort. I owe a great deal to Bill Cole of Peterson's. Without Bill's encouragement, the project would still be in the planning stages. Rick Cowan and Heather Hoerle of NAIS Boarding Schools deserve a thank you for their initiative in asking me to speak at the 1992 NAIS Conference in San Francisco. The conference provided fertile turf for coordinating a strong team of writers and gave us the opportunity to brainstorm as a group.

A special note of appreciation goes to Roland Barth of the Harvard Graduate School of Education whose "Teacher as Leader" concept inspired me to finish *Casualties of Privilege* and begin *Healthy Choices, Healthy Schools*. Ted Mitchell, Rich Maxon and John Rassias, my mentors, have long recognized the link between affect and cognition and helped build my conviction that students cannot realize their full intellectual potential without a strong base of self-confidence and healthy relationships.

I appreciate the leadership shown by Deirdre Ling of Middlesex School, Malcolm Gauld of Hyde School, Susan Graham of The Gunnery, Chris Horgan of Dublin School, Lawrence Becker of Brooks School, Dan Heischman of the Council for Religion in Independent Schools, and Bobbie McDonnel of Phillips Academy, who openly recognized *Casualties of Privilege* as an important tool for professional development. I would be remiss not to recognize the valuable assistance of John Koch of *The Boston Globe*, Sharon Basco of Monitor Radio, Marty Nemko of "School Talk" NPR in San Francisco, Robert Forbes, Linda Fosburg, Dan Brewster, Mary Dunn, Marcia Schaeffer and others whose interest in honest evaluation and school improvement bolstered the success of *Casualties of Privilege* and lay the groundwork for *Healthy Choices, Healthy Schools*.

On the editorial side, special thanks to Robert N. Pyle & Associates for providing office space and equipment, Chris Crowley whose valuable work established Avocus' distribution network, Ernest Peter for his good ideas, humor and fine business sense, Kelley Busby and Ted MacVeagh for their literary and legal insight, Jennifer Peter for her editorial advice, and Karen Klunk for her proof-reading. Of course, the biggest thank you of all goes to Claire.

Contents

Preface

Casualties of Privilege: Essays on Prep Schools' Hidden Culture, the first book in Avocus' boarding school series, sparked considerable reaction in the prep school world. From comments like "I deplore 'casualties of privilege' on account of the general sweep of its implications, as a phrase and a book, that would tar the vast majority of bright, sensitive, well-meaning, conscientious, supportive, and hard-working members of our community . . ." (Charles H. Clark, Rector, St. Paul's School) to "Crosier's book is a call for honest self-assessment. I urge all boarding faculty to read it," (Bill Cole, Peterson's), the book started an important dialogue about the health of residential programs.

Since its publication, more than 60 percent of NAIS boarding schools have purchased *Casualties of Privilege* and 8 percent of prep schools have bought in bulk for the professional development of faculty, parents committees and trustees. *Casualties of Privilege* has been used in workshops and conferences including the NAIS Heads' summer symposium and Peterson's national workshop series. Mr. Crosier's related speaking engagements include the 1992 NAIS conference in San Francisco, the New England Association of Independent School Librarians Spring Meeting, the Independent Schools of Northern New England Dean's Conference and individual school seminars. Mr. Crosier will lead a panel discussion on the link between affect and cognition at the Educational Records Bureau Conference in October 1992.

Healthy Choices, Healthy Schools is the sequel to *Casualties of Privilege*. Its goal is to advance the discussion on improving residential life. The book will structure the questions raised in *Casualties of Privilege* and serve as an initial clearinghouse for solutions to these problems. It will help schools identify what systems might be in place to provide a healthy residential experience for both students and faculty and will allow individual institutions to determine where they stand in setting up those systems.

While *Healthy Choices, Healthy Schools* will discuss "what works" and strategies for implementation, the book is intended as a point of departure for dialogue between schools, rather than an end in itself. Since each school possesses unique circumstances and a distinct mission, each will determine what systems are best suited to its particular needs. At the 1992 NAIS Conference it was exciting to see heads, deans and faculty from all over the United States talk about differences in the way their schools operate and solve problems. *Healthy Choices, Healthy Schools* will build on these productive conference sessions.

Healthy Choices, Healthy Schools does not exhaust the topics of concern to modern boarding schools. Notably absent are AIDS, hazing, adolescent sexuality, raising your own children in the dorm, and retirement. Although many of the systems described in the book relate to these issues, they do not deal with them directly. I hope future books will include these important topics.

Avocus Publishing, Inc. produces group-authored books on timely social issues. Our goal is to encourage meaningful dialogue and promote healthy choices and responsible behavior. If you would like to contribute to one of Avocus' forthcoming books or would like to coordinate a book project, please contact the Avocus office at 202/333-8190.

Mark Baker, Vice President
Avocus Publishing, Inc.

Foreword

by Louis M. Crosier

Individual Improvement

The key ingredient in professional development is honesty. Without honesty we cannot identify what needs improvement. We live in a culture supported by an infrastructure of passive lies. Advertisements bombard us daily with distorted images of what it takes to "look good" and "be happy." Our kids' heros are often less desirable and less real than we might hope: the Terminator, Wayne and Garth, Joe Isuzu. Politicians rework their vocabulary and leverage the events of the day to create smoke screens and disguise their past. Growing up in this environment, we learn to fib and eventually tell a full-blown lie. Let's call it "marketing mentality." In order to sell a product we must believe it is great. Sometimes we have to trick ourselves to cover up its weaknesses. But if the people in research and development thought the product could get no better, we would soon be out of business. The same is true for schools. In external affairs— admissions, development and often the head's office—schools get better results if they believe 100 percent in their product. However, internal positions— faculty and deans—can be more realistic. Here honesty is essential. In order to provide our students with the healthiest learning experience we, as educators, must acknowledge our weaknesses. That, in turn, will improve the product and benefit enrollment, retention rates and annual and capital giving.

It's not surprising that many teenagers lie to their parents. In addition to a social climate which appears to reward the most artful dodgers, students lie because the consequences they associate with the truth often threaten their tenure at school. They lie to avoid letting themselves or their role models down. Lying allows them to break the rules and maintain other people's respect in the short run. Unfortunately, they lose in the end. First, they do not benefit from an open relationship with a role model who could provide needed advice; second, they do not address their potentially self-destructive behavior; finally, they risk the consequences when their behavior and the lie ultimately surface.

I think teachers and parents often promote lying because they are reluctant to discuss uncomfortable issues. Take the case of the parents who do not want to believe their sexually active child may not be a virgin at 14 or 15 and may have already risked exposure to the HIV virus. By avoiding discussing the issue with their child, not only is the child having intercourse but he or she is doing so without a parent to turn to for advice. This child might also be lying to avoid

3

disappointing the parents or receiving a punishment, and the lie further compounds the issue. Similarly we often find excuses to avoid dealing with our shortcomings in the classroom or residence hall. Lack of time and resources, the universal scapegoat, takes the blame for our mistakes and keeps us from addressing the issue: how can we get better at what we do?

We all know people who are excellent "brown nosers"—the kind of person who can nod convincingly when he doesn't understand a word you're saying. This kind of "pretending" gets us surprisingly far in the short run, but ultimately catches up. We do not necessarily get caught, but further down the road we figure out we have built much of our lives on appearances with little real substance. We don't know very much and realize life would be more fulfilling if we did. But the older we get, the harder it is to admit what we don't know. So rather than ask questions, we often build a strong facade or avoid unfamiliar topics.

On the other hand, many of us are honest about what we need to improve but are resigned to leave it alone and continue what we do best. But "you can't teach an old dog new tricks" is an unacceptable attitude for teachers—of course you can, it just takes more bones. For example, part of the cause of continued adult illiteracy is the embarrassment of admitting it. We need to create a climate in our schools which makes it OK to admit what we don't know or when something isn't working. Another example: Why are we reluctant to endorse national teachers' exams? Are they insulting? Will we fail? Will they raise standards? What's to fear? And what kind of message do we send students: "We won't take tests, but you have to." Wouldn't studying for these tests and passing have a positive impact on teacher confidence which would transfer to the classroom? I believe a good test which covered a subject area, some adolescent psychology, and basic teaching theory would do just that. Over time the wrinkles would work their way out of the exam and schools would enjoy a higher standard of professionalism.

I have never been very good at history. I read nearly as slowly as I speak. Memorizing dates is "impossible." But when I moved to Washington, D.C. last September I was suddenly surrounded by people who knew about the presidents, the wars, and the U.S. political system. In short, it was awful. I found myself getting shut out of many conversations. So I began reading about individuals who had played a role in government—a few dates and a lot of detail. I visited the National Portrait Gallery—it's free. After a few months, I surprised myself in a couple of conversations. Although I didn't dare say anything, I could follow along for the first time. Now I will tentatively offer a comment here and there. I'm still learning and people are more receptive to my comments than I anticipated. What an incredible boost of confidence for someone who had resigned himself to being a mediocre history student!

There is a risk when jumping into unknown territory, but it is certainly worth it. If we create a supportive atmosphere in our schools and among faculty members, we can go a long way toward improving our teaching in and out of the classroom. As teachers we need to do more of what we are asking of our students: we need to become active learners again. Seeing us try, sometimes fail, but always get back up sends a strong message to kids and colleagues about the road to success and our determination to get there.

In the fall of 1989 I took Eleanor Duckworth's "Teaching and Learning" course at the Harvard Graduate School of Education. The class showed me that very intelligent people often don't know simple things. I discovered that my classmates and I all learned differently and that the "smartest" people were the ones who asked the most questions and pursued them until they got the answer that made sense. Then they would take an extra minute to try the answer out to make sure it worked, just like a young child. Kids learn fast because they are curious; they ask endless questions. A wonderful cartoon in the *New Yorker* magazine shows a man holding a small boy by the hand. The child, looking up wide-eyed, points to the clouds above. The man says: "That's a cloud too, they're all clouds." As teachers we have experienced this many times. The child explores, discovers and tests repeatedly to find permutations and verify accuracy. In order to improve our schools we need to relearn the basic skill of asking uninhibited questions until we understand, then trying out the answers, continually refining as we go.

Since the release of *Casualties of Privilege* I have received praise and criticism. The praise keeps me going and the criticism fires me up to work harder on improving my work and the effectiveness of my delivery. The headline of a recent article in the Dartmouth College newspaper read: "Crosier '87 Shines in Publishing in Dismal Times." The article began by exaggerating my success in these recessionary times. Then, toward the end, a passage read: "Last term, Crosier was a guest lecturer for 'The Private School' a course offered by Dartmouth's education department. . . According to some of the students, Crosier was not a particularly impressive speaker. . . ." What? Outrageous! Since then I have been asking people I respect what they feel it takes to be a good speaker and have restructured my speaking style accordingly. The book itself received extreme reviews on both sides. Most widely criticized was my methodology, and most highly praised was my honesty. The exciting part of feedback spanning the whole spectrum has been the opportunity to take an honest look at what I have done and see what stands up to repeated scrutiny. I am able to refine my recommendations with each new piece of advice and continually ask myself questions to improve my weaknesses. Much like a course I took in college where the students had to rewrite each paper until it met a certain standard, I have benefitted from reworking the same thoughts up, down, and sideways, again and again. A beneficial parallel can be drawn between this exercise and our work as teachers.

Collective Improvement

Just as we begin by taking an honest look at ourselves on the individual level, we must do the same on an ongoing basis on the institutional level. We need to identify the necessary components of a healthy residential environment. Then we can determine from a broad list what systems we have in place to ensure we meet the standards we set for ourselves.

Schools have elaborate systems even if they aren't labeled as such. All schools have a system for discipline, for rooming, course selection, assigning advisors, counseling and running the dorms. These systems vary from school to school and we can benefit from finding out how other schools do it. Collectively, schools can begin to arrive at composite pictures of what works best. That's a big part of what this book is about. For example, variables in the discipline system from school to school include: second chance vs. first offense expulsion; composition of the Discipline Committee—faculty only vs. faculty and students; a committee which makes decisions vs. a committee which makes a recommendation to the head or assistant head. There are almost as many systems for discipline as there are schools, but they all fall under the category of discipline. It was fascinating to work with a group of fifty deans, heads and faculty at the 1992 NAIS convention to discuss how they might improve their systems. Some of the most valuable exchanges involved representatives from schools whose systems were polar opposites. There were deans whose schools subscribed to the triple threat, a great way to work with students in multiple contexts, and others whose schools felt strongly that "separate" residential faculty, whose sole function was running the dorm, should be the structure of choice. This provided the opportunity for representatives from differing models to take a look at the benefits of each system, to identify overlap, and to see how their problems differed. Through discussion they made suggestions about how each might strengthen their programs without major structural change. One dean asked of another: "How do you handle rooming?" He went on, "We have always had trouble ensuring our younger students finish their homework and get enough sleep." The other responded: "We handle that problem by housing our freshmen and sophomores in singles and our upperclassmen in doubles." Another hand went up. "How many of you let your students go in the dorms during the day?" Most schools did, but some did not, and a discussion about liability as well as unity between day students and boarders ensued. The process was eye-opening because it became clear that we often feel stuck in one of our systems, even though the first step toward an answer may be as simple as a few phone calls to other schools.

Most schools have sophisticated systems for handling the standard issues of residential life. But few have systems for handling the intangible side: a system for assuring that all students make friends; a system to ensure that all students get enough sleep and eat healthily; a system to ensure adult presence. An important part of the health of a residential environment lies in its intangible systems.

Once we identify all the systems we believe our school needs, we should look at where we stand in the evolution of each system. Some are relatively new (Gay/Lesbian) and we are ironing out the bumps. Others have existed for a while but may not have been used much yet (AIDS). Others have been fully operational for a long time and refined repeatedly. Finally, we have systems which have existed since the founding of the school but which have not changed to reflect the times. After identifying the systems that need work, we should talk with people at other schools to see how they handle the same issues. Sometimes we do this on a local level, but rarely do we seek advice on a national level. We should. Schools often struggle unsuccessfully with an issue for months while another school in a different part of the country has an effective program in place for handling it. After collecting information about alternative systems, faculty and administrators should pursue the discussion within the school.

As systems evolve we should poke holes in them to see how they stand up in different situations. Too often we allow a crisis to arise before we see how our system responds. Alternatively, we could run the system through a series of hypothetical scenarios before the crises occur. As we refine our systems we need to combat the hurdles of complacency and staleness among our colleagues. The best way to guard against these is to keep an ongoing program of professional development, including individual role play, group scenario work, and conference and in-service training.

Healthy Choices, Healthy Schools takes a close look at existing residential systems highlighting "great ideas." Several of the essays provide an historical perspective tracing a school's evolution on a particular issue. These chapters are important because they demonstrate evolution through refinement. Each essay brings a unique perspective to the discussion and each contributor takes the initiative to suggest ways we could be better at our jobs, proving we can all be leaders.

Collectively, independent schools have extraordinary resources for problem solving. I hope this anthology will help us look at age- old challenges in new ways. *Healthy Choices, Healthy Schools* is meant for educators at all stages in their careers. Whether you are new to the profession, deciding whether or not to make it a career, or dedicated to residential education as a way of life, the essays herein should spark new ideas to make your job easier. I hope the book helps you work together with colleagues and students to make healthy choices and improve the quality of residential life at your school.

1

Connecting with Kids: Boarding Schools rather than boarding Schools

by Bill Poirot & Dusty Richard
Brooks School
North Andover, Massachusetts

Casualties of Privilege raised some crucial issues for boarding schools and especially for faculty who have dormitory responsibilities. Some of the stories represent our worst fears: the student who feels uncared about; another who sees dorm parents as the enemy and the institution's impact as essentially confining and negative. Those of us who choose to live with the kids hope to have a different kind of effect on their time at a boarding school, and hopefully on their lives.

Boarding schools do not differ from the great day schools, both private and public, in the quality of the intellectual experience. By whatever measurement you choose to employ, some of both will be found at the top of the list. Nor do boarding schools stand out based upon the variety or the excellence of experiences available outside the classroom. Outstanding student newspapers, ambitious outdoor clubs, and nationally recruited athletes are found at both kinds of institutions, and the excellence of the offerings is not determined by whether the kids go home at night. Clearly what distinguishes boarding schools from equally strong day schools is the fact that the children live together. That is our greatest opportunity for enhancing the education they might receive at a day school; it is also our greatest challenge.

Certainly the stories of *Casualties of Privilege*, for the most part, catalogue our failures, at least with the individual students who wrote of those experiences. Parents who had not had previous experience with a boarding school would certainly not be inclined to spend extra money to assure their children of that set of memories. On the other hand, families who have for generations sent their children to boarding schools, as well as those parents whose first child to attend had a positive experience, know something not readily understood from reading *Casualties of Privilege*, and many have voted with their checkbooks to repeat the experience.

Most families have at least one of three fairly simple reasons for considering boarding school. The first has to do with the child. He or she may be bright and bored, bright and lazy, average but ambitious, highly talented, easily distracted, or lost in the crowd. Many of these are reasons to consider independent schools in general rather than boarding schools in particular. However, such descriptions of the child are often coupled with a family situation or an aspect of the current living environment which suggests a change. The family situation may be as simple as both spouses working, both traveling for business, or it may be a complicated divorce or another type of one-parent household whose nurturing capability has been stretched too thin. The family may simply want someone to be "home" for the child after school hours. Some parents feel that only-children are particularly well served by boarding schools. Finally, the home environment may be wrong for the child: too dangerous, too remote without companions, or full of childhood friends who are not headed in the parents' preferred direction for their child. Schools in the area may lack racial diversity, may have too narrow a band of extracurricular opportunities, or may overemphasize athletics. The adolescent culture in the town may be excessively materialistic or shallow.

Student, family, environment: boarding schools can offer necessary corrections to a perceived imbalance in any or all of these, because the school choice is not bound by geography. The children at a given school will be of the same age and roughly of the same academic ability, but they can be from radically different cultures, climates, backgrounds and circumstances. They will almost certainly have startlingly different preparation, values and expectations. And they will have a group of adults who have chosen to live among them. Dorm parents are not saints, although the best ones approach that category. Some are strict, some are more flexible, they all make mistakes and they all get weary. But they all choose to live with the kids, to get into the middle of the growing process. That process cannot help but be enhanced by the listening, the hand-holding, the disciplining, and the values clash which comes from that interaction. This is the heart of the boarding school promise: that some adult will become involved in the life of each child, will come to care about that child's growth and development, and that the caring will make a difference in the child's education.

Boarding school offers parents a group of adults who, as ill-advised and rash as the decision may appear to the rest of the world, have chosen to live with children, night and day, inextricably bound up with their young lives, willingly susceptible to the disappointments and triumphs, the betrayal and loyalty, and the constant intensity of the adolescent world. Children who grow up in boarding school cannot avoid all non-academic contact with adults; they cannot hide in the numbing conformity so often demanded by the adolescent culture. Most, despite what they say and how they may act, do not want to avoid all contact. They do want to check themselves against some authority, however ancient and decrepit, measure their growth against some yardstick, however suspect in their group. During a period of dizzying change in their lives they need someone to be a stable center, someone to take a role between the unconditional love of their parents, which is not reassuring and can be stultifying, and the harsh judgment of the world. From the adults who choose to live with them they need something less than the love of their parents, and more than the simple task demands of their classroom teachers. They need to feel a concern emanating from their dorm parents, essentially positive and hopeful, accompanied by some expectations and demands which are inseparable from a genuine caring. The fact that the adults choose to live with them is almost enough by itself. They will accept strictness, they will forgive weakness—although they will undoubtedly exploit it—and they will readily include you in their lives.

The relationship between a dorm parent and a student can be a very powerful force for good. It can motivate the student to grow in ways that are important to the adult world, such as becoming better organized, more responsible, and a higher achiever. It can also encourage the children to develop in ways that are meaningful to them. They can become more skillful at relationships with their peers, practice leading others, discover the flexibility within themselves which is necessary for successful living with others. Sometimes the relationship can help children value themselves in ways that head off self-destructive excesses of behavior which shocked us in *Casualties of Privilege*. The relationship is not guaranteed to moderate the behavior of those cared about, but it may be the best hope. It is at the very least an agreement on the part of students to be answerable to the ones who care about them. They may pause, reconsider, even back off from some planned activity because of their relationship with a caring adult who has chosen to live with them. If they were always that thoughtful, that rational, of course they would not be adolescents. They will let down the caring adults, and hopefully they will reflect on that.

Most schools think carefully about who is assigned to dormitory duty, and perhaps even how such duty is perceived within the school. The older model is being replaced by new thinking. Gone, hopefully, are the days when the newest teachers went into dorms where they acquired sufficient experience and expertise to be effective at about the same time as they accumulated enough seniority to get out of dorm duty. More schools are matching the energetic younger faculty members to older, experienced faculty families. In some schools effective dormitory supervision is seen as a professional accomplishment on a par with effective teaching or coaching. In such institutions it is acknowledged, rewarded, and even honored explicitly. Dormitory parents have an important voice in crucial decisions about the running of the school. They are upper level administrators, department chairs, and are seen within the community as valuable resources. Perhaps the easiest way to understand the value that a school places on its residential life is to see what else at school the dorm parents do.

It was amusing for veteran faculty to try to identify the schools involved in the stories from *Casualties of Privilege*. Some schools could be identified with certainty, others with a high degree of probability from some of the details. What became very clear was that the stories were told about some of the finest boarding schools in the country. I suppose by "finest" I mean hardest to get into, and "containing the brightest students as measured by their standardized testing." Faculty at such schools seem to me particularly susceptible to the belief that what distinguishes them from other schools for parents are their high academic standards of which they are appropriately proud. Such schools may place a great deal of weight on the classroom performance of its teachers, and perhaps value less the dormitory responsibility. The objectivity and rigor so necessary in the classroom, the detachment, may come to be seen as virtues in the running of dormitories. Relationships formed around the performance of tasks and the subsequent evaluation of that performance become the normative standard. One is suspect if he or she is seen as being too close to the kids. In such schools the most respected faculty members will have nothing to do with the dormitories. They will live in big houses on the edge of campus or off campus. The senior administrators will, by definition, not have to do dorm duty. The dorms may be seen as the place where you warehouse the students from the end of classes one day to the beginning of instruction on the next.

All boarding schools try to create an enhanced learning atmosphere. Some are able to gather exclusively students of superior ability, in which case the drive of such students is enough by itself to insure a serious academic environment. Most concentrate unusually heavy resources of time, money and human beings on the education of a relatively few. All create a structure which has proven to be effective in maximizing the performance of each student. The promise then for the enrolled children is that they have been placed on the fast track, been given an unusually rich opportunity to become educated. Their responsibility in this contract is to take the fullest possible advantage of these opportunities. The price they pay is the forfeiture of part of their childhood. They must give up free time, the chance to follow idle curiosity, the chance to play without responsibility. They must adopt adult ways of dealing with time, organize themselves around tasks in emulation of the most successful adults, and follow a rigidly proscribed pattern of intellectual inquiry and daily routine. Most do not want to do this. Many acquiesce. Some rebel with all their hearts. It is not at all unusual for the fiercest of the rebels to be among the most intelligent, the most thoughtful of the group.

In many ways the most selective schools have the greatest challenge in their dormitories. The adults may be assigned to live with the students rather than choose to do so. Their responsibility in this respect may have considerably less value, less prestige in their faculty community. The children may be the most self-aware of their generation, having figured out what they are giving up and what they are getting. They do not in their hearts accept the trade off, and they are angry. Angry at their parents and at the school which so callously strips them of their childhood pleasures. They may be assigned to the dormitory randomly, or in pairs, or other combinations of small numbers. Thus their loyalties are first to their peers, and may never extend to the adults who in some cases are "on duty" only every eight nights. Should we be surprised when these students act out their anger by outwitting the junior varsity (in their eyes) faculty members assigned to be their keepers? Is it any wonder that they see the rules, designed at such schools to minimize the interaction between adults and children, as appropriate targets for flaunting as dramatically and on as wide a scale as possible, as an almost inevitable focus of their anger?

No school is going to completely escape experimentation of limits by adolescents. On the other hand, a dormitory living arrangement characterized by concern on the part of the adults for the children, can help them care for each other and for themselves. If the adults get in the habit of listening, they will hear when the kids are worried about themselves or about others in the building. You can create an atmosphere of caring about each other in a non-sentimental, non-judgmental way. The model is not so much a family as a small town, where you acknowledge some responsibility for each other, where you might scold a neighbor's child who is playing with matches, or take your neighbor's sheets in from the clothesline when it begins to rain. The children in a dorm ought to be chosen for an existing relationship with one of the adults. They could be students whom dorm parent advises, teaches, coaches or supervises in an activity of interest to both of them. I believe those children should remain under the care of that same adult as long as they are at the school, or until they wish to try a dormitory where they have another adult with whom they have a relationship. Adults should ask for students in their dorms on the same basis, and when the school gets to the last five kids to be assigned rooms, it will know who is in most need of connecting with an adult. The school will know with whom it needs to renew the boarding school promise of having a caring adult involved in the education of each student. The school will know where to direct its energies and resources in order to cut down on the *Casualties of Privilege*.

* * * * * *

Immediately a new cycle begins. In the academic sphere the succession of tasks is formal, highly organized, and increasingly complex or abstract. The evaluation component often provides an individual with the core of his or her standing in the school and, in many cases, a corresponding self-esteem. The athletic arena sets a simple task, preparing for the contest, and the evaluation is equally simple, almost binary: win or lose, on or off, one or zero. The better coaches know what the best teachers have always known, that the real lessons, the genuine excitement, and the lasting self-esteem come from the preparation phase rather than the evaluation. Even in the extracurricular life of a school, which is usually organized voluntarily around shared interests, some task and the evaluation of its performance is usually at the center of the group's activity. How do we judge what kind of year the band had, or the drama group, the French Club, or the Student Council?

Schools are about tasks, performance and evaluation. All schools. Children learn how to be reliable, punctual, accurate and thorough in the performance of their assigned task, and at the higher end, self-starting, thoughtful and even creative. The reward for learning to perform tasks well is high evaluation and subsequent placement in a more able group at the next higher level of tasks. In this context, which all schools share, dormitories are an anomaly. In the first place only boarding schools need concern themselves with the living arrangements of their children. Let us for the moment concede the now almost universally accepted hypothesis that college students are adults, not children, and that the universities need only assure them of some place to live, without adult supervision and without responsibility for the quality of those arrangements beyond what is required by law of any landlord. I've often wondered why the colleges, perhaps under the influence of the marketers, have vigorously replaced the word "dormitory" with the expression "residence halls." Is it because the word "dormitory" suggests adult presence?

When we think or talk about "school" in this country, we are not concerned with dormitories. If we recorded all the conversations in the faculty rooms across the country, all the meetings in schools, in communities, the meetings of professional organizations grouped by discipline or by administrative position, what percentage of those conversations would be about dormitories for high school age students? One percent? No more than three percent. Is it any wonder, then, that boarding schools fall into the trap of seeing the dormitory component of their operation as peripheral? A cynical colleague of mine once characterized the non-dorm teachers' view of dormitories as, "a place where you warehouse the students until they are scheduled to appear again in my classroom." The comment suggests that most day teachers (those who do not share responsibility for a dormitory), if they think at all about dormitory life, think about it in terms of control. Yes, we are a boarding school, and, yes, the children live right here where they take their classes. Of course we must provide them with a carefully supervised place to study, see to it that they get a decent amount of sleep, and that the stronger ones do not pick on the weaker ones; in effect, we must maximize our chances of having an optimal encounter with each student in class the next day. When dormitories are discussed by the whole faculty, it is almost always one of these control issues which precipitated the discussion.

I am suggesting that even in most boarding schools, the issue of dormitory life is not central to the school's self image. The faculty in most boarding schools are divided on the subject and I am afraid that, even among the dormitory parents, only a few see their work as absolutely central to the worth of the school. School is school. Academics are at the core of any school's existence. They define the school and give it its value in the marketplace. Athletics and extracurricular activities can add value to the core, but dormitories are like the food service, or the snow removal or the building maintenance: essential that they be done, but not essential to the quality of the educational experience. You could get a great education even if the food was terrible.

Perceptive dorm parents have always known that, in fact, their area was at the core of the school experience for adolescents. Their former charges have come back ten, 20, 30 years later and told them so. They have known it instinctively from their first day living with the children, and they have behaved as though it were true, stealing time and emotional energy from their other duties and pouring them into dorm life. They know that the impact on the children is enormous, almost as great as the rewards and satisfaction flowing into their own lives. They have not pressed their case on their colleagues largely because they suspect that it would fall on deaf ears and, besides, they want to keep the goodies for themselves.

The institutions, on the other hand, were slow to hear the message, for there were no external pressures on them to change a formula which had worked for centuries. As the demographic times became tough, however, admission directors began to talk to the rest of the administrators about the quality of the food as a recruiting tool. Gradually the facilities arms race expanded to include dormitories, although many boarding schools have buildings which offer them little flexibility on this issue, short of wholesale gutting and remodeling. An impressive athletic complex, library, or arts center is still a more important recruiting device than the dormitory rooms. So while the dormitory buildings may be no higher than fourth on the list, at least they have now made the list. Once schools began to discuss the qualities of dormitory buildings, a discussion of the quality of the experience going on in those buildings was close behind.

In the old days—not the good old days, just the old days—parents used to entrust their children to a boarding school. They took their direction on the raising of adolescents from the school, and the school undertook more than just the academic education of their charges. Besides Latin and algebra, schools agreed to provide a moral education, instruction in manners and hygiene, a physical education which emphasized teamwork as well as *mens sana in corpore sano*, help in developing daily habits which would allow them to become productive students and later adults, and finally guidance of their interaction with each other with an eye toward nurturing, at the very least, good citizens and hopefully leaders. When they dropped off their children the parents quite literally backed off, "let go" in the current idiom.

Today's parents as a group have more trouble letting go, and in fact frequently stay in close, even daily, contact with their children. This need to micro-manage their children's lives has brought the current generation of parents into much closer contact with the daily life of the school. Can anyone who taught in a boarding school in the 50s or 60s imagine a Parents' Committee? This juxtaposition of the traditional role of the boarding school and of the current parenting style suggests two clear implications: one, that those parents are certainly going to press the school to deliver on the promise of a complete education, especially at prevailing tuition levels; and, second, that they are going to focus more of their attention on the residential life of their children. And they may well do so with the dormitory parents as their first line of approach.

I am suggesting that residential life in general and the dormitories in particular are going to be the next frontier for independent boarding schools. A recent survey done for real estate professionals pointed out quite convincingly that parents are no longer looking for the best/hardest school they can get their children into. Instead they are looking for schools where their children can be successful, where they can be challenged and stretched without being driven or worn out by the competitive atmosphere. Certainly the brightest boarding candidates, the ones who are also ambitious at age thirteen, will continue to group themselves at a handful of the most selective boarding schools in the country. But even those schools are going to be in competition with one another for who can provide the most supportive and healthy residential side of the equation.

I recently sat in a room full of educational consultants, people who work closely with families in finding the right school for their children. They told the group that parents were no longer going to send their children to schools which were rigidly inflexible, hung up on their academic standards to the point where they were callously harmful to children. Some quite prestigious schools were included in that description, along with their gentler but equally distinguished competitors. The rest of the boarding families in this country, some with children equally bright but less ambitious, others with children of average intelligence, will be looking for a healthy, growth-producing experience at a school with the right academic challenge for their child.

If the promise of a boarding school is that one of the adults will connect with each student, then dormitory life will provide at least as many, if not more, chances than the classroom or the fields. For the latter are essentially task-oriented, and that task will usually establish the basis for a relationship. The essential task of the dormitory is for the residents to live in harmony with each other for the school year. Yes, you must clean your room, be quiet during study hours, and check in on time, but these checkpoints are neither the primary nor the only basis for a relationship. When it is working at its best, a dormitory can feel very much like a large family, a place where everyone has a separate agenda, but where all respect each other, gain something from interaction and even develop various levels of affection for the people with whom they are living. If you are a boarding school person who thinks that this is pie-in-the-sky idealism, ask your graduates who their closest friends from school are, and which are their most pleasurable memories.

Boarding schools ought to pay a great deal more attention to their dormitories than they have in the past. Such a process might begin with an internal audit comparing the time, energy, resources, and thought which goes into the dormitory life as compared with the academic.

- Are dorm parents as a group scheduled to meet as frequently as the full faculty or academic departments?
- How is dorm responsibility weighed against teaching load?
- Are the channels for dorm parent input to the running of the school comparable to those established for teachers?
- How much of the faculty development effort (budget, professional days, conferences, summer courses) goes to dorm issues?
- Does the school set aside any time in the daily or yearly calendar for dorm issues?
- Does the daily or yearly schedule favor non-dorm faculty?
- Is some of the housing most sought after by senior faculty attached to dorms?

The audit might continue with a look at the weight placed on dormitory work in the hiring and then the advancement of faculty members in a boarding school.

- Are dormitory skills considered in the hiring process, and what weight are they given compared to teaching and coaching?
- Does the school ever recruit a star dorm parent as it might a department chair or head coach?
- Are teachers ever recruited with the explicit understanding that they will not be required to do dormitory duty?
- Is dormitory work included in the evaluation process, and is it given weight comparable to the time expected to be devoted to it?
- Is successful dorm parenting one of the skills which can move a teacher into an administrative position?

The surest way to know an institution's position on dormitory responsibility is to examine the question of status within that institution.

- Does the culture of the school recognize superior dorm work in the same ways it recognizes superior teaching?
- Are the dorms staffed essentially by younger faculty?
- Does the school culture encourage staying in or moving out of the dorm?
- Can a faculty member avoid dorm work and remain at the school in a way which would be impossible if it were teaching being avoided?
- Can an inept or disinterested dorm parent carry on when a similarly inept or disinterested teacher could not?

- Does the institutional culture encourage top level administrators to remain in a dorm as vigorously as it might encourage them to continue teaching?
- Are top level administrators exempt from dorm duty?

I suspect that faculty in boarding school will always be hired by academic departments, with an appended list of what else they might do at the school. That seems appropriate and naturally efficient. The question is not whether dormitory work is second or even third on the job description, but rather how close a second or third, or whether it is on the list at all. I think every school is beginning to pay greater and more careful attention to staffing the dormitories with faculty who will do as good a job in that role as they do in teaching their academic subjects.

If my brother asked me how to evaluate the dormitories at several boarding schools he was considering for his child, I would first tell him to determine the experience level of the dorm parents. When a school can keep long term faculty happy in its dorms, then that aspect of the faculty member's work is rewarding in a way that must be good for kids. When that group of long term faculty still in dorms includes several top level administrators, then you are looking at a school which is in touch with its dorm life, enables and values those who work in dorms, and grants them status.

The best dorms are run by compatible teams of adults, working together in a harmony which models the behavior they expect of the student residents. I think it is very much worth the institution's time and trouble to carefully build such teams, even when that team-building takes considerable effort and intricate interpersonal balancing. The team must work together or the battle for the goodwill of the kids is lost before it begins.

The team must include some parent types, people with experience raising children. Veteran faculty who have seen generations of students through adolescence certainly qualify as parent types. The point is for parents to meet someone whom they immediately (and subsequently) feel confident will provide substitute parenting for their children. The team should also include someone young enough for the students to relate to, and with enough energy to keep up with them—judgment from the older dorm parents and energy from the younger. If either party has both, then so much the better.

If the school is serious about finding a way for each child to connect with an adult, then the ratio ought not to make such connecting unlikely or impossible. One adult for every ten or 12 kids seems reasonable. Faculty spouses who are happily involved in the dorm life may certainly be counted, but not those who remain apart. The residents will quickly tell you which is which. Long before I would remodel the student rooms in a large dormitory, I would knock out some walls, put in kitchens and bathrooms, and increase the number of faculty living in that building. Interns and beginning faculty are great in such situations, as long as they are paired with older, experienced, parent types, and are given some direction and mentoring. Adolescents draw a great deal of energy from their environment; they are almost an emotional black hole, and young teachers can supply enormous quantities of that required energy.

The school's method of placing students in the various dormitories will also be highly revealing of the institution's thinking on the residential life. Several years ago one school used to require all the students to move twice in a school year so that they lived in three different places during that time, hardly a scheme to encourage the connection between dorm parents and residents. The model which makes the most sense to me is one in which the dorm parent teams are established for the following year, then student leaders of each building are invited to serve under adults they respect and with whom they already have a relationship. Finally the students are invited to list their preferred order of housing. Priority is given first to those already living in a building, on the assumption that their choice to remain suggests an existing relationship with one of the adults. Then the older students are given priority over the younger ones, and the dorm parents have some input based on their connection with the individual students seeking to live in their dorms. Kids who are particularly difficult to live with are quickly identified in this process and can be distributed evenly among those dorm parents who feel they have the best chance of reaching each individual.

The danger, of course, is that dorms can begin to seem typed, usually around the personalities or interests of the presiding adults. I'm not sure this is bad, as it is a natural consequence of basing the housing decision upon relationships made in other areas of school life. If all the wrestlers live in the wrestling coach's dorm, it is only going to be noticed in the winter season. If all set design students want to live in the stage manager's dorm, is that not a reasonable and decent principle upon which to choose one's living arrangements? Furthermore the rewards may far outweigh the dangers, for dorm parents who work closely with students in some other capacity have far greater natural leverage with their residents. A student must literally think twice before letting down not only his/her dorm parent, but also his/her teacher . . . coach . . . activity director. Advisors should have priority in bringing their advisees into their own buildings. In fact, the negative side of the natural tendency for students to gather in groups is actually mitigated when the organizing principle for dorm selection is the relationship between the dorm parent and each individual student.

If no relationship is expected of the dorm parent, if it is in no way part of the institutional expectation that they will connect with the students in their building, then any number of methods of assigning students to rooms are appropriate. Lotteries, for example, are fair in the sense that they are impartial. On the other hand they are highly impersonal; perfectly appropriate for colleges, less so for boarding schools. If connecting is part of the plan, then almost any relationship is better than a lottery. The strongest connections tend to be between advisor and advisee, then from the classroom, athletics or activities, then such considerations as older siblings with whom the dorm parent connected previously. Sometimes a student and an adult can come together for no other reason than that one or the other of them senses that a relationship might form. Even that hope, the potential for a relationship, is a better reason to put a student in a particular building with a certain adult, than the spin of the lottery wheel. Schools with large dormitories can use the house system to encourage the kind of connections more easily made in smaller dorms.

Dormitory life distinguishes boarding schools from other options. Schools where the children live together cost as much as a third more than day schools, and parents are beginning to take a closer look at what they are getting for that premium. Internally, schools are looking at the educational possibilities for the dormitories, as opposed to seeing them simply as warehouses. Neither colleges, day schools nor high schools face these challenges, and boarding schools have only recently begun to consider the active educational role dorms might be capable of playing. So the discussion is going to be both new and confined to a fraction of the educational community. Those schools which create the most supportive, healthy atmosphere in their dormitories are likely to gain a competitive edge on the ones who see all dormitory issues as simple ones of control—check in on time, be quiet during study hours, clean up your room, and don't pick on the younger ones. The dormitory offers schools a great opportunity to teach getting-along-with-other-people skills, which are going to be required in most colleges and highly sought after in the work force of the twenty-first century.

2

Let the Four Horsemen Ride

by James T. Adams, Assistant Head
The Lawrenceville School
Lawrenceville, New Jersey

Casualties of Privilege, not surprisingly, caused a bit of a stir in the world of private boarding schools. These are perilous times for such schools, demographically and financially, and it is unsettling when you are wondering how to survive to be asked to wonder whether you ought to. But before the NAIS, like some secular Gideons, sneaks the book with its ten commandments ("Ten Steps Forward") into every dean's desk, let me make three simple observations: 1) sixteen disaffected voices given the charge of articulating their particular laments forcefully enough to merit inclusion in the volume should not be presumed to speak authoritatively for the experience of hundreds of thousands of other "prep" school students; 2) much of what they described is hardly peculiar to boarding schools; and 3) many of them concluded by saying something akin to Hibbard Melville's final summation: "My experience there was invaluable." In other words, if this is the worst that can be mustered against the industry, we needn't wonder whether we ought to survive.

All this is not to say that the book itself shouldn't survive, and I hope a lot of deans find the thing in their desks and read it closely. Students do sometimes fall through the cracks at boarding schools, and when they do, they have been more than failed; they have been betrayed. For the *raison d'etre* of any boarding school that can justify its tuition has to be that its residential program offers a worthwhile educational adjunct to its curriculum that is responsive to the needs of every student whose parents believed that when they enrolled him in the first place. So it is well that *Casualties of Privilege* sounds the alarm about these potential betrayals, and it is especially appropriate for the book to conclude with quite specific suggestions that might redress the apparent problems. Indeed, I subscribe wholeheartedly to Mr. Crosier's decalogue, "Ten Steps Forward."

He believed, however, that these steps will constitute the "time dividend" of

20

redefining the residential faculty role so that "boarding faculty should begin the day just before dinner" because "parental duties take precedence over academic responsibilities." I reject this notion out of hand for several reasons.

First, starting the work day "just before dinner" simulates babysitting, not parenting. Parents of adolescents do not roll out of bed at 5 p.m. Rather, typically, they have full days themselves before resuming their parenting responsibilities. If their exhaustion undermines their "quality time" with their children, its causes offer compensatory benefits. Adolescence is a time when children are groping towards a sense of self independent of their parents, when in fact overly attentive parents might suffocate this awkward but natural and important development in their children's lives. The business of learning to perceive oneself as an entity independent of one's parents, capable of making important decisions on one's own, should be encouraged by the child's concomitant discovery that his parents have lives independent of his. Children do not make a successful transition to responsible adulthood if they do not understand that their right to increasing independence must be attended by the revelation that the sun does not revolve around them anymore. Increased independence uncoupled with increased responsibility and self-reliance is a delusive and dangerous species of freedom indeed.

Adolescents are not adults, to be sure, but they have a powerful need to spit the bit. To change the metaphor, there comes a time when the training wheels must come off the bike. Parents should perform this chore, not the children. There will be some harrowing accidents and it's better to get them out of the way in the fenced-off yard of prep school than on the busy street of real life. The parent who is fresh enough to run along side the bike forever isn't doing his child much of a service. To abandon metaphor altogether: we must free adolescents to meet our adult expectations of them, and then, because they are not adults, must be there instantly to forgive, to advise and to support even as we let them suffer the consequences of their failure.

Secondly, I think it's time we scrapped the term "dorm parent." We aren't their parents and they don't want us to be. In fact, for the very reasons cited above, adolescents are probably better served by adult role models other than their parents as they navigate the uncharted waters of their emerging adulthood. They already have parents, most of them loving and supportive, and in my ten years running a house of forty boys, I met very few Holden Caulfields who felt abandoned by their parents just because they weren't under the same roof. Anyone who has run a dorm with any degree of rapport with his charges knows that boys and girls confide things to their dormmasters that they wouldn't to their parents, and they will frequently respond instantly to advice offered by the dormmaster that Mom or Dad has offered with abject futility a million times before—and they respond to it exactly because it is not their parents offering it. It is much easier for students to discern the objective wisdom of adult guidance if it is not charged with a lifetime of parent-child emotional electricity powering any number of agenda at once. The time is fast approaching in their lives when they will not be obliged to respect parental authority, but will be obliged to respect other authority figures. Adolescence is the ideal time to get used to that development, and boarding school is, or can be, an ideal place for it.

Finally, what kids don't need is a highly energized pseudo-parent counseling them madly about aspects of their lives that are perforce abstractions because his day has just started and he's never seen the kid in the classroom, in the locker-room, or in the hall between periods. That dormmaster must depend upon the "book" for his counsel, not his experience with the individual. Students know that, and their parents are paying a pretty penny to help them avoid it. If I learned anything from my decade in the house, it's that you don't really know students until you've known them in a variety of contexts—and the same goes for their knowledge of you. Once they've seen you hold forth in the classroom, throw your clipboard on the playing field, make time for your own children, as well as roam the halls in your underwear after lights out, well, then they know you; and the comprehensiveness of your knowledge of each other is the first prerequisite for the intimacy that will beget, not only the most effective, but also the most rewarding teacher-student relationships possible. Everyone, students and faculty alike, wears a variety of hats, but it is not sufficient merely to know that; the dormmaster must see them tried on before he can appraise the fit.

So if the fresh, specialized surrogate parent isn't the answer, what is? I still give the nod to the exhausted "triple threat." Exhaustion is a handicap, I grant you, but I submit it is not the source of the deficiencies detailed in *Casualties of Privilege*. In fact, I recommend laying considerably more responsibility on the dormmaster.

The Four Horsemen of the Apocalypse, as far as dormmasters are concerned, are Exhaustion, Frustration, Guilt and Anxiety; and they are foes to be reckoned with. But they are the inevitable concomitants of commitment and caring, and you cannot easily mitigate the former without vitiating the latter.

Students need and deserve commitment and caring from their dormmasters, and I believe they are more likely to receive it—and, incidentally, to give it—if they can look to one adult, the one they bump into around the clock, for just about everything and if the dormmaster quite understands and embraces that overwhelming responsibility. To have one dean address the student's brushes with the law, another monitor his academic progress, somebody else advise him with course selection and yet another specialized counselor who can't know him as well as his dormmaster assume responsibility for his painful progress through adolescence, etc, is to draw and quarter the student intellectually and emotionally, to leave the professional who knows him best in the dark, and to give the parents too many phone numbers to call. Kids need mentors, not advisory committees.

Nobody ever loved an advisory committee. But the bond created between a teacher and student who instinctively find each other and no one else when some crisis, any crisis, erupts in the student's life can be a powerful one indeed. When the bond is there, the student's little failures or the dormmaster's lapses have decidedly human consequences that are not merely recorded, but felt. When the relationship is more human than official, its obligations are more moral than legal; and when a student senses a moral obligation, a few implicit expectations will accomplish much more than a raft of explicit rules; and when he is thus warmly enveloped by benign moral expectations and not straight-jacketed by arbitrary regulations, that is, when he is expected to be good and not bad, chances are he will respond because he owes it to the faith of his dormmaster.

The issue, and it's surprisingly subtle, is trust. Today's post-Vietnam, post-Watergate, post-Ivan Boesky kids are wisely chary of extending it to any adult authority who hasn't proven himself worthy. Some degree of intimacy is a prerequisite to that trust, and in the absence of trust, that is, in the absence of the sort of intimacy described above, the real if unavowed first purpose of a school's residential program becomes behavioral control, not moral empowerment.

You catch more flies with honey than with vinegar. A school's residential program should appeal to a young person's best instincts— they fairly riot inchoate within him—and equip him to identify them, organize them, hone them and finally use them himself to combat his selfish impulses, which likewise are live and well in his character. If a school focuses its energy in some puritanical way on the repression of his base instincts, if the student is too heavily burdened by some oppressive sense of his Original Sin, the best the institution can achieve is to abet the dubious maturation of a person whose loftiest aspiration in life will be to fight a kind of moral holding action, and who will forgive himself readily for failing even in this because he has become cynical of his own and his fellows' capacity for inviolate decency and altruistic intention. Believe a student is good, make him believe it, and he will one day be less ready to forgive his own moral shortcomings than those who believed in him, and this because they believed in him. You give him the confidence to explore the best that is in him and the will to turn it to some humane and serviceable end because he will believe that others, like himself, are worth the best he can muster.

When we fail to achieve the intimacy that will beget this trust, we must restrain the child because he will see no reason to restrain himself. This is how student underground subcultures are formed. To return to an earlier metaphor, if we refuse to remove the training wheels from the bike, band-aids at the ready, the students will take them off at night and ride in the dark.

Here's my advice for what it's worth: decentralize your residential program. Make the dormmaster the headmaster of his house and get out of his way. Instead of herniating to find ways to subdue the Four Horsemen running him down, make his job so important, so worthwhile and rewarding that he'll scarcely notice he's being trampled. Help him, or her, foster intense identity between the student and his house. Let dormmasters develop unique traditions, perhaps field their own intramural teams, do things as a house instead of as a class. Make the kid's house feel like a home and let him know who's head of the household. "Home," says Robert Frost, "is where, if you have to go there, they have to take you in." Kids should feel "taken in." Alienated kids develop subcultures and alienated dormmasters hear thundering hooves. In sum, students and dormmasters have to be in it together, and they have to be in it wholesale. Let the Four Horsemen ride; June is on the way.

* * * * * *

What follows is a description of a working model of the philosophy described above. As I am an alumnus of Lawrenceville as well as a former housemaster of ten years service, I can be justly accused of bias in asserting that our house system is a unique strength of The Lawrenceville School, but I hope any school rethinking its residential program will give serious consideration to our arrangements.

Lawrenceville's house system has three levels, Lower School for eighth and ninth graders, Upper for our seniors, and what we call Circle Houses for our sophomores and juniors. Because whatever virtues our house system has are most clearly reflected at the Circle level, I'll limit my description to that for the sake of brevity.

Each Circle House, and we have ten (four for girls, six for boys), has 30 boarders and approximately 15 day students associated with it. Typically the housemaster is married with children, and he or she works closely with a live-in assistant, typically young and single. Other faculty, called associate housemasters, will take some duty nights, attending to check-in, etc., and, in fact, the housemaster is formally "on duty" only two nights a week, one of which is always Saturday night. Practically speaking, of course, the housemaster is "on duty" anytime he or she is in the house.

The housemaster is given extraordinary responsibility and discretion. He or she is the student's academic advisor, counselor of first resort, surrogate parent, disciplinarian, friend, frequently the coach of one of the house teams, and perhaps the classroom teacher of his charge, certainly his tutor of an evening.

Our house system, curiously enough, mirrors the federalism of our nation in that the house (states) generate their own rules, and breaches of these rules are adjudicated internally. There are, of course, federal laws concerning drinking, etc., that will involve the dean of students, but each housemaster is free to govern his fief as strictly or as loosely as he deems appropriate. It is not unusual for neighboring houses to have radically different television policies or study hour rules.

Houses tend naturally to take on something of the character of the housemaster and each house is perceived to have a collective individuality in which students take great pride. Each boy or girl, no matter now strict his or her housemaster, is likely to believe his or her house is the best. The collective individuality is encouraged symbolically. Each house has its own colors and flag, and each has developed unique traditions. Only alumni of Cleve House, for example, are allowed to use a certain entrance to the house; the boys presently in residence are obliged to use a less convenient one. House pictures from years gone by are hung all over the place, as are plaques commemorating this or that. Each house has its own awards and trophies. Each has its own duly- elected council, and depending of course on the housemaster, the house president can be a powerful force indeed.

Each house has its own dining room in our central underform dining center; and while no rule obliges students to eat in their own dining rooms, they inevitably do. Each house fields its own intramural team to compete against the others (the hundredth anniversary of Circle House tackle football was recently celebrated on ESPN).

Houses frequently hold dances or take field trips; they have Christmas and year-end banquets, thrice weekly coffee hours and Saturday night "feeds." In short, the student's social life revolves primarily around his house, which gives a large school the inflection of a much more personal and intimate place.

Students are sharply identified with their house. No list of students (or alumni for that matter) or classroom roster is ever published that does not list the student's house, and because all faculty know who is housemaster of each house, all faculty know from day one who their students' advisors are. That makes communication between teacher and advisor commonplace and natural. In addition, our house mail system allows for nearly instantaneous written communication between teachers and housemasters or students. If, for example, a student fails a French quiz in the morning, his housemaster will know it that night, as a yellow academic progress slip, known by students as a "canary," will arrive in the mail that evening. If a student surprises a teacher with an A on a test, that same canary will bear the good news just as efficiently, only now it is called an "eagle." Similarly, any class absences are discussed the evening of the same day.

The consequence of all this is that the housemaster is inevitably on top of all aspects of his charge's life and parents need call only the housemaster to get the whole scoop on junior's progress. Relationships between parents and housemasters are frequently as powerful as those between housemaster and student, and as likely to endure. Indeed, the housemaster *is* Lawrenceville as far as the typical boarding parent is concerned.

Because the housemaster is everything to the students of his house, his is a high stress job that requires as much patience as energy. The strain shows. A few years ago we held a late summer conference on housemastering to explore ways to relieve the stress and increase job satisfaction. What we discovered, paradoxically, is that the sources of stress were also the prime springs of satisfaction; that is, the overwhelming responsibility of the job is simultaneously its boon and bane. Apparently there is marginally more boon than bane here, for vehemently as housemasters clamor for relief, even more vehemently they denounce any erosion of their responsibilities. In other words, they like their jobs. They must: the average tenure of housemasters is about eight years, the average age of our Circle housemasters is over 40, and recently two housemasters who had done long stints in a house returned to housemastering. Lawrenceville has yet to suffer the problem apparently epidemic in the rest of the secondary school world: a dearth of willing housemaster prospects. This is especially significant in that we demand so much more of our housemasters than other schools.

When so much responsibility is reposed in one individual, it behooves the school to reward that individual, and housemasters benefit from a subtle range of perquisites that cumulatively enhance their remuneration substantially. Their apartments, especially in the older houses, tend to be enormous and well-maintained (of course at no cost to the housemaster). Though there is no formal policy that says so, housemasters tend to get larger salary increments than other faculty. In a curious vestigial gesture that harkens back to the days when house dining rooms were actually in the house, our dining center delivers breakfast groceries—eggs, milk, coffee, bread, juice, etc.—to the housemaster each week for his own use. When housemasters of significant tenure retire from the house, they go right to the top of the list for desirable campus housing.

One of the expectations of our current capital campaign is to improve housemaster compensation even more. We are seeking to endow housemastership, which should enhance both the salary and prestige of the position, and we intend to offer housemasters special honoraria: ten percent of the average salary of our faculty will be set aside annually into an escrow account where it will compound quietly until a housemaster of seven years service or longer retires and claims it. That bonus coupled with the school's generous faculty mortgage plan should allow retiring housemasters to buy a second home.

Speaking of retiring housemasters, I should close with the following anecdote. Recently a couple retired from housemastering after 36 years in the same house. Alumni of their house organized themselves and gave them a send-off that I believe would not have happened anywhere else. They bought the couple a condominium in Florida, a trip around the nation and a variety of other gifts. I do not believe a more centralized residential program in which housemasters are relieved of primary responsibility for nearly all aspects of the child's life could ever generate the affection and loyalty that resulted in that generosity—or in the honored couple's pride in their career. Our housemasters are in it with the kids, and they are in it wholesale. That makes the real difference.

3

Getting A Life: The Challenge of Self-Care to Adults in Boarding Schools

by Daniel R. Heischman, Executive Director
The Council for Religion in Independent Schools

. . . facts are kept alive by being told, logic by being demonstrated, truth by being professed.

Erik Erikson, *Insight and Responsibility*

But as caring for another engrosses me in the other and redirects my motivational energy, so caring for my ethical self commits me to struggle toward the other through clouds of doubt, aversion, and apathy.

Nell Noddings, *Caring*

''Get a life'' is one of the more frequent expressions heard on the lips of independent school students around the country. Like similar injunctions, such as, ''Lighten up,'' or, ''Get real,'' it is designed, like other commandments in different contexts, to tell others how to live, and to express how we feel about the present nature of their personalities and dispositions.

Presumptuous as it may be, ''Get a life,'' can also be a defense, a reaction to the perceived presence of others judging us or expressing concern about us. In that way, it is a means of holding on to one's present attitude. Rather than allow someone else's viewpoint, values, to have any relevance to the character and content of our own lives, we, along with our students, respond by accusing the other of having nothing better to do than meddle in our own affairs. Back off, and get a life—your own!—so that you can stop looking over my shoulder.

It doesn't take much to realize that such phrases are reflections of the need for adolescents to feel some control over their own lives, to have privacy, autonomy, and protection from the watchful eyes of adults or their peers. If nothing else, the very articulation of the words themselves, put together in a catchy and contemporary phrase, betray the need of adolescents for some sense of power over the worlds they inhabit. Nonetheless, there is some truth, even some wisdom in this defensive posturing, something which all of us who work with young people need to be reminded of from time to time. We adults do, indeed, need to get a life!

Moreover, the key to a healthy environment in a school community has to do not only with the happiness and productivity of students, but also the sense of fulfillment experienced by the adults who work daily with those students. As Nell Noddings concludes, "A school cannot care directly. A school cannot be engrossed in anyone or anything. But a school can be deliberately designed to support caring and caring individuals, and this is what an ethic of caring suggests should be done."[1]

In another context, I have expressed my views on the helpful, as well as the questionable, contributions and perspectives to be found in the volume of essays, *Casualties of Privilege*.[2] Among those essays, the most memorable, and worthy of further reflection, was the one on "Depression," written under the name of Frederick Connolly. At a couple of instances in the essay, the writer speaks of the teachers he encountered in his boarding school, and noted that the work demands they contended with, as well as the 24 hour nature of the job, made them seem as "stuck," as permanently in residence at the "Hotel California," as any of their students. Consequently, they shared the plight of the students they taught:

> It seemed like I was living in a children's environment. Even the "grown-ups" acted like kids—they were as unstable as we were . . . The teachers were role models, yet we knew they were overextended: teaching, dorm-parenting, and sometimes coaching (the "triple-threat"). It seemed as if they were as out of control as we were.[3]

Depressed by his own situation in school, the young man seems similarly despondent by a lack of hope he senses in the lives of those adults around him. His cause for concern for the teachers he encountered should stand as a reminder to all of us in the adult world: when, in our style of life or in our outlook on life, we begin to "mesh" with those whom we are there to help, then we're in trouble, and we have lost our crucial, critical distance.

It seems to be part of the nature of the adolescent to seek seemingly contradictory goals in life: independence, yet authority; autonomy, yet limitations and boundaries; stability, yet flexibility; freedom from adult interference, yet the assuring presence of adults. At times the young person seems to be asking for both simultaneously, exhibiting the fact that young people can be, ". . . both cops and robbers, cowboys and horse thieves—alternately but passionately."[4] It is a confusing world to comprehend, let alone enter into and work with on a daily basis.

When it comes to the adults with whom students at boarding schools interact on an intensive, daily basis, the same kind of contradictory expectations come into play. On the one hand, the young person prizes the caring presence of adults whose outlook on life and practical values are accessible, thoroughly human, in some way a reflection of who he is as well as what he wants to be in life. In the presence of such adults, the adolescent can observe and comprehend, and in some way see reflected in that life himself or herself at a future point.

At the same time, the adolescent seeks an adult who embodies the "other," something over and above the values and perspectives of the youthful world. Be it the adult's wisdom, experience, exemplary character, or passionate commitments and convictions, the student can see in this adult a person calling himself or herself to be something more. As much as an adolescent might appreciate the ability of a teacher to enter into the world of youthful humor, if that is all the teacher seems capable of doing, the young person remains ultimately dissatisfied. All of us know of instances in which students who initially valued and looked up to the young teacher who seemed to mirror much of what they, as students, experienced in life, found themselves, over a period of time, uneasy with that teacher's lack of adult perspective. To sustain the trust of an adolescent, there must be, in the adult, a sense that the values and experiences embodied in that adult are not something which, in a very short period of time, the young person is likely to outgrow.

In short, the young person needs to experience both a confirmation of his present identity as well as hope that he can transcend the conflicts and confusions of the adolescent world. The adult offers both empathy and hope, confirmation and challenge, and only this difficult but essential combination is worthy of the adolescent's trust in the midst of the conflicting needs that characterize this stage of life.

The above is hardly news to most of us who work in schools. What it may serve to do, however, is remind us of the dual nature of schools: to attend, on the one hand, to the needs and growth of students, as well as, on the other hand, to nurture the adults in the community who are guiding those young people. No students in our institutions will benefit from an educational environment that is excessively student-centered; it is in the interest of our students that we acknowledge and foster the healthy development of the adults in the community, who, in turn, will offer the hope that is necessary for the well-being of those students. In a world in which the line of demarcation between the adult and the child is increasingly porous, a healthy picture of adult life is all the more—not less—important.

A wise and experienced teacher recently remarked, in the midst of a faculty meeting, that schools are institutions where many people are engaged in a process of finding themselves, and not all of those people, he reminded us, are students. This is true of the young teacher, who recently completed college or graduate school, whose tireless energy and boundless enthusiasm is both a blessing as well as an essential ingredient for the ongoing operation of a boarding school. That teacher, whose chronological age may be quite close to that of the students he or she guides, may very well be viewing the academy as a place of reflection and self-discovery, a context in which he or she can consider what career options may be most desirable. The school is clearly grateful for and dependent on his or her ability to work arduously long hours. Are there healthy ways it can also acknowledge and appreciate the personal searching that characterizes the life of the young adult? This is also true of the veteran teacher, who has devoted many long and enviable years to our institution, but now is growing older. Gradually that teacher may begin to discover that he or she may not be able to keep up with the herculean pace of younger peers on the faculty. Are there ways we can benefit from the veteran's accumulated wisdom and loyalty to the school, while affording that person the opportunity for a less demanding pace of life? Are there options in the life and work in the community more conducive to diminished energies?

The adults in a school community must, in other words, be engaged in the process of "getting a life," and securing it in ways that are important to their respective stage in life. As obvious as this may seem, we need to be reminded of it continually lest we overlook the disservice we do to students by not attending to the needs of adults in our school communities, and lest we forget that the process of identification, on the part of young people toward adults, is as essential to the educational process as books and learning.

In Richard Ford's novel, *The Sportswriter*, Walter says to Frank Bascombe, "When we get to be adults we all of a sudden become the thing viewed, not the viewer anymore."[5] To my mind, implicit in that comment is as sound a view of adulthood as one could find: the awareness that one has passed over into a new realm, where one is being watched, observed, noted for one's reactions, one's distinctiveness over and above the world of the student. If for no other reason than the fact that one is being so thoroughly and—at times—critically viewed, the adult becomes aware that he has something to give, that he has an awesome duty in the midst of a learning community.

As I work with faculties throughout the country, I am impressed by their extraordinary commitment, compassion, sheer ability to sustain a level of energy and caring and good humor, not to mention love of their work, in institutions which are increasingly demanding and pressurized places in which to work. What does concern me, however, is the tendency of good people, such as faculty members, to deny their own needs, discount the fact that their well-being figures into the well-being of their students. When such neglect sets in, we are prone to being more critical of our students, less in touch with our colleagues, unmindful of our friends outside of school or at risk in our relationship with our family and spouse. We as adults not only suffer, the entire community feels the lack of breadth and liveliness in the lives of its adults.

Frequently, I will help faculty consider the moral climate of their schools, and I am both touched by their concern for the integrity of their students and concerned, at times, by their reluctance to draw themselves as adults into the picture. In those instances, morality becomes a matter of single-minded focus "on the kids," what they are or are not doing, or what their parents do or do not stand for as they raise their children. Some of that, of course, may be our natural human reluctance to implicate ourselves morally, in any way. But it is also a means of shortchanging ourselves and the importance we play, the power we have, in the lives of young people. To my mind, the moral values of a school begin with what the adults in that community hold dear, how they treat each other as colleagues, how they are aware of the nature of their conversations with and about their students. If it does not begin there, it must, at least, necessarily end up there. As one teacher remarked, there is a "boomerang" quality to our discussions about the moral environment of a school: we may begin by talking about our students, but the issue always, always comes back to us.

I am tremendously impressed with the progress I have seen in many schools in building up programs for faculty development and enhancement of opportunities for further study. Some school heads or deans of faculty have an uncanny ability, in gestures of appreciation or expressions of concern toward faculty, to attend to the person behind the intellect. Many leaders of our institutions have gone unheralded for their concerted (and courageous, in the face of budget-minded trustees!) efforts to raise faculty salaries, one of the most eloquent testimonies to the visionary and big-hearted character of these caring people. Faculty retreats have become increasingly important ways that teachers can draw upon their insight and wisdom as adults, as well as experience a sense that they are valued as professionals. Guest speakers, such as Sarah Levine and Peggy McIntosh, both of whom stress the value of being in touch with our inner lives, our inner resources, encourage faculties to form ongoing groups as a means of staying in touch with each other as colleagues. I am frequently reminded of some words I heard Peggy McIntosh say, in response to the question of where do we begin to value and understand multiculturalism; her response was to be reawakened to and draw upon the multicultural within ourselves as adults.[6] As a result, our schools are increasingly places in which our adults can thrive, as human beings and as guides to young people.

Still, the pace of institutional life is quickening, not languishing. I have seen more faces of fatigue, among faculties, this past year than in previous years, not to mention heard more concern expressed by faculty about the lack of time—how they feel cut off from their colleagues by the demands of their routine. Time—this most precious of modern commodities—is an increasingly important issue among our teachers, and, as I remember Peggy McIntosh explaining to me on the same occasion as above, time becomes an urgent issue when we are not clear about what we are doing or why we are doing what we do. Opportunities for one of the most valued of all faculty activities, interaction among colleagues, is perceived to be increasingly rare. In order for us to avoid the perception, let alone the reality, that our teachers are just "as trapped" as our students, our creative powers will need to be directed toward the means by which we can further enhance the adult lives of those on whom our students so depend.

I think we are coming to a point in the lives of our schools when we are going to need to structure informal reading time, not only for students but also for adults. Test scores are increasingly indicating that young people are doing less and less reading outside of the classroom, so the setting of actual periods of reading may become, for our students, a pedagogical necessity. For adults, on the other hand, the setting of reading time—be it on an individualized basis or through reading groups—may be yet one more way to acknowledge the human need for and the professional importance of our faculty members to maintain full reading lives apart from their work.

Furthermore, as insurance premiums continue to rise, I would encourage schools to fight to maintain provisions, within their health plan, for faculty to make use of mental health practitioners. I find it ironic that, at a time when we are frequently expanding our counseling services for students, we are tempted to trim the mental health benefits for the adults in the school community, who are similarly experiencing increasing levels of stress and fewer opportunities for self-renewal and self-reflection. Good therapy always stresses the differentiation of self from those with whom one works, and that is clearly a necessary mode of operation in the intensity of boarding school life.

When I was in seminary, I remember reading a newspaper article by the English writer, Monica Furlong, bemoaning how her local vicar, on whom she relied heavily for spiritual support and nourishment, was all too tempted by the hectic character of the modern world. As Ms. Furlong concluded, "I do not wish my priest to be a fellow competitor in the rat race of the world." The truth of that desire has implications for our students and their development, as well as the well-being of this priesthood we call the teaching profession: young people, in their search for credible adults in whom they can trust and with whom they can identify, do not need mere mirrors of their own experience. They need people who have "gotten a life," a life different from, and calling them to grow beyond, the world of the adolescent; they people whose values are worthy of imitation and whose personal fulfillment offers them hope for the adult years which lie ahead of them. As tempting as it is to focus on young people in our work, the ethical and emotional well-being of adults is the key to a future which is open and hopeful to youth. "For whoever wants to cure or guide, must understand. . ."[7]

Notes

1. Nell Noddings, *Caring: A Feminine Approach to Ethics and Moral Education*, page 182.

2. See, "Casualties and Challenges", *CRIS Newsletter* (September 1991), page 1.

3. *Casualties of Privilege*, page 61.

4. Erik Erikson, *A Way of Looking at Things*, page 627.

5. Richard Ford, *The Sportswriter*, page 185.

6. These were remarks made by Peggy McIntosh, at a general session of the annual conference of the Independent Schools Association of the Central States, November, 1991.

7. Erikson, *Identity, Youth, and Crisis*, page 137.

4

Teachers Who Are Parents: Different Priorities At Dublin School

by Andrew J. Brescia
Dublin School
Dublin, New Hampshire

If all our sons or daughters are really as special as Mister Rogers says they are, then why do some parents choose boarding schools the way they choose a car? Why are they shopping for the right "look" or brand name and the sticker in the back window announcing that the "baby on board" is growing up at a school everyone knows will open college doors?

These parents know full well that schools do mold their students, despite Holden Caulfield's assertion to the contrary in *The Catcher in the Rye*. The molding, after all, is what the colleges recognize when they admit students from those prestigious schools like my own alma mater, Phillips Academy. Those "top" schools mold a student who strives for the only kind of success some parents (and many colleges) seem to understand or value. Those schools do indeed open doors and are justifiably proud of graduating "tomorrow's leaders" in every conceivable profession.

As much as I credit larger schools for succeeding in their mission, I believe now that they can learn something from what a small school like Dublin can do better.

More Than Just Opening Doors

At Dublin School we believe—from the headmaster down—that the around-the-clock education our boarding school should offer depends on trust and healthy relationships more than how many national merit semi-finalists are harvested out of each junior class. We think it should have less to do with how many of our students take AP exams in May than whether we instill in our students an understanding of community that people can really only talk about at larger schools. Understandably, then, you will not find the college counselor's office next door to the headmaster's. In fact, you won't find one at all. Instead, each of the 25 or so returning juniors can choose one of six faculty or staff members who serve as college counselors. Teachers at Dublin can greet all students by name after a few weeks of classes, and, by the year's end, we know more about each one of them than many teachers at larger schools know about their "advisees." All teenage students, after all, need more than high standards, wherever they are, and students at Dublin are offered much more.

At Dublin we believe that a boarding school's education can recommend a lifestyle not primarily concerned with achievement-driven success.

The classroom education at boarding schools is as good as the questions students of varied abilities feel comfortable asking. Extraordinarily low teacher-student ratios can help if, like any other advantage, the teachers and students capitalize on the opportunities those advantages provide. But if the teachers are good, their students will learn (at any school) how much more they can learn from good questions than from knowing the "right" answer. Their teachers, in the meantime, will continue to ask their own good questions for students to better understand how to make familiar, one question at a time, what once seemed unfamiliar.

Those questions become the means to an end in each and every classroom. They become a kind of "style" of learning for students of all abilities and levels of enthusiasm, and, if they feel successful, or begin to personally acknowledge the benefits of good questions, they will be the students in college who write more questions in the margins of their textbooks, notebooks, library books (in pencil), and even on their desks if they have to. And it won't stop when they graduate, we hope.

In all boarding schools, though, the questions don't stop when class is over. The proverbial "playing field" is a place for questions, too—only students in small boarding schools have an edge over teenagers elsewhere.

The afternoon is a time to ask questions about when to crowd the opposing goalkeeper who's a bit on the short side, how to push the lefty over to expose her weak backhand or how to keep the scouted senior with a great finishing kick from winning yet another race. But it invariably becomes the time, too, for the "coach" to ask questions about a student's previous evening in the dorm, family pressures, or why that student is not letting up at all during practice, day after day. With every afternoon's van ride and athletic contest the students-turned-athletes learn, we hope, that the victory often goes to those who troubleshoot and critique with different kinds of questions internalized from hours of good coaching or talking. The "ya gotta want it" stuff gets them only so far.

Teachers might have two or three students each year they really click with. Coaches often have that Pele-like striker or Jim Ryan run-alike around whom they can build a team, as well as those athletes guaranteed to win most improved honors at the all-school awards ceremony. Teachers who also coach can have both, and at a small schools like ours there will be more than one or two. Those teacher-coaches will click in one way or another with most of the also-rans, too, with those whose moment of fame may be finishing sixtieth (instead of sixty-eighth) out of 70 runners or making the one clumsy assist that wins the game. At Dublin those teenagers will, by their senior years, more than likely be scoring off those assists and placing in the top twenty in a league championship! But for that to happen we work at treating each member of our teams as important—in practice and during contests—by emphasizing as coaches that all our students participate.

It's at the small schools of less than 200 students where teachers who teach with questions and coach with questions—and a loud whistle or merciless stopwatch—can also impersonate Oscar the Grouch or Mister Rogers in the dorm for many of the same teenagers. And when the dorm, more properly called a house, beds between ten and 20 teenagers, those teachers can become parents who learn, year by year, how to ask the better questions that those teenagers need to answer: about why trusting anyone is difficult, why familiarity is good but intimacy is difficult, or if living with the consequences of our actions might actually mean living with an identity formed by the choices we grow up making.

At its best, Dublin School is such a school. I have taught and coached a boy here who lost both parents to suicide. I have taught a boy who went from being a freshman with an "attitude" to an honor-roll junior with enough reason to believe in himself that he began standing up in all-school assemblies when he felt compelled to defend doing the "right thing." I taught, coached, and lived with a sophomore whose older brother was the closest thing he had to a father, and by his senior year he was swelling our hearts with pride with his words and deeds. None of these graduates has all the answers, but we don't expect them to. Like the rest of us, they are still asking questions about who they are and how they belong.

Students everywhere wrestle with their own questions, but our teachers and students agree that at a small school like ours availability and familiarity help us earn their precious trust. They are then willing to ask some more questions to enable some of the pieces of their lives to begin to fall into place. None of them grew up next door to Fred Rogers or Bert or Ernie, although some begin by pretending they have. Pretending, in fact, is clearly near the top of the list of strategies for both the well-groomed teenage drug dealer I lived with ten years ago and the "girl" who has already appeared on the cover of *Seventeen* but is a recovering anorexic. Pretending is how comfortable roles slowly become indistinguishable from an identity and every teenager's private goal: happiness. Pretending, however, is not the stuff honest and trusting relationships are made of. It is instead a recipe for dysfunction later in life.

In Loco Parentis

Sooner or later it becomes clear to teachers who coach and live at schools like Dublin that living with teenagers *in loco parentis* does not mean they are ever merely dorm supervisors, study hall monitors, classroom teachers, or members of a coaching staff. It does not really mean they have office hours or "off-duty" nights. What it means is that they have a house full of children who are all being teenagers at the same time and who will, like any house full of children, have as many different needs as there are moods in a day. It means going *loco* sometimes trying to teach, coach, and live with a group of human beings who are, in the words of one counselor I know, at the most emotionally promiscuous stage in their lives. Sooner or later, it becomes clear that *in loco parentis* means what it says. Teachers at Dublin become parents, for all practical and immediate purposes. Oscar or Fred, take your pick.

At small schools the around-the-clock education can seem stifling to the students and too much of a good thing to the teachers. It often exhausts even the most vital and resourceful faculty, but it means helping the also-rans better understand how to find the way to their own happiness in addition to passing the next algebra test. At small schools, because of persistence and an ever-growing familiarity with our students, we can help them participate more actively in their lives and develop an ever-increasing autonomy until they learn to do both. At larger schools those kids—whose personal lives and conflicts remain largely a secret—will too often be told just to work harder.

Some students don't make it. Some aren't ready for that much attention and find a way to leave; others, despite the support, can't swim academically or emotionally. Some Dublin students may even find a crack to hide in and, like students at larger schools, seem remarkably impervious to the influence of teachers, coaches, and their boarding-school parents. In fact it is good for some to do just that because they are already focused and participating in their own lives by making decisions without seeming to be distracted by "issues" besieging their classmates. They seem to be making good choices and are on track, and some are. Those students invariably become senior proctors on whom we rely to do their own share of advising, guiding, and attentive listening. They, too, are rarely "off duty" at Dublin.

Others, however, are simply excluding themselves—as they have learned to do without giving offense or taking any—from many of the relationships available to them in what is more like a true community than I have seen at either of my other two schools (approximately 600 students) or in my own experience at boarding school.

It's tempting for the *loco* parents to pity those who exclude themselves and miss opportunities, but perhaps the sentiment badly disguised as pity expresses our belief that the child in each of us learns more about how we define our own happiness from relationships, open and trusting, than from believing that "good fences make good neighbors." It's tempting, too, to shake our heads like so many dashboard basset hounds when we faculty talk about some of the parents our students trust about as much as their parents trust them. But neither the pity nor the "parent bashing" has a place in the curriculum at any school whose teachers hope to educate their students and themselves with questions that help to resolve conflict and heal relationships. Besides, more than a few of our parents already have trusting relationships with their teens.

For those who step over the cracks—and later look for cracks to fill in—a school like ours becomes a place where it's safe to talk about all those things that fell off the shelf inside and shattered into so many pieces. All children, by the way, have something to talk about. There needn't have been a death or divorce in the family for a child to feel hurt and alone; it may be something as seemingly benign as a little neglect. It's even safe in our classroom discussions to read between the lines of the chauvinist's poem or the anorexic's short story. Even the sophomore who could be at Andover discovers why his teenage ;protagonist, feeling distant and ignored, is sitting in the back seat when both his parents fall asleep at the wheel. Our students feel safe discussing these topics and gaining insight into their lives as soon as they know we are listening because we care. They learn quickly that it is our agenda at Dublin to care about how they understand and resolve conflict in their lives. Isn't this kind of insight and self-knowledge, after all, one of the most practical results of the much-acclaimed "critical thinking?"

In classes of ten students (often smaller!) it's easy for students, again, to become teenagers—or even kids—who are not too busy developing those critical thinking skills to begin seeing why they haven't felt as special as Mister Rogers insisted, gently, that they were. Ditto, of course, for the "dorm" of 12 or the tennis, squash, cycling, or sailing team with just enough players to compete officially.

In fact, if we are to believe what a number of Dublin seniors tell me, it is the "dorm" more often than not that provides the time and place for the growing familiarity between our students and residential faculty to pay off in the conversations culminating in many a "momentary stay against confusion," to quote Robert Frost.

The Sense of Security

Run by only two dorm parents, our small dorms at Dublin begin by providing what all boarding school dorms offer: that limited autonomy a teenager enjoys in being away from home. "You're on your own, away from your parents," one senior told me, "but not really." Most teenagers in boarding school can enjoy that after the initial and often recurring periods of homesickness.

But dorms at Dublin also define a daily routine for our students by becoming—primarily because of the presence the teachers establish from day to day—more than a place to "crash" after another day's work. Supervised evening study halls at Dublin mean a faculty member who is visible throughout the evening, popping in and out of rooms and doing his or her own reading in the dorm's common room or apartment—with the door open. An enforced lights out rule means a dorm parent and/or proctor standing in doorways until the light goes off (and checking later, too). Dorm parents and proctors also share the responsibility of supervising (and helping with) the daily cleaning jobs and room inspections. All this defines a routine of obligations and accountability to both senior proctors and dorm parents. This routine helps students define their own responsibilities, focuses their attention and energies on community life and helps them feel more integrated into the life of those around them.

"Lewis," a day-student-turned-boarder, points out that suddenly teachers and students were available to him throughout the day and evening. His growing familiarity with adults came from having them stop in to chat on the edge of his bed or sit in the dorm commons and try their luck at the latest video game. It came from being perceived and feeling he belonged and was finally "involved." Dorm life at Dublin redefined for him the categories of adult relationships available to him —from the headmaster, who he says was the first to believe in him, to the classroom teachers, coaches, and dorm parents. Even though every teenager will agree it's easier to associate with students than adults, it is equally clear to Lewis that teachers who foster a teenager's sense of autonomy, by listening without compromising the expectations of the school community, will change a teenager's all-important perceptions of the role of adults in his or her life.

Finally, Lewis adds, teenagers will rely on the "helper" who respects, supports, and trusts as well as the "enforcer" who sets the limits by imposing the structure and routine. For "Marie," another day-student-turned-boarder, the dorm life, with 11 other teenage "sisters," replaced the isolation of living at home and provided her with two "elders" in dorm parents which seemed "like having other relatives to communicate with"—older friends whose reactions to her questions she need not brace herself to hear. Neither the listening nor the discipline of dorm life, it seems, will have much substantive effect without adults who are genuinely interested in parenting.

"Bernard": A Case Study

If anyone epitomizes what Dublin can teach a teenager through relationships, "Bernard" does.

Described as a "pimply, gangly, gee-whiz" freshman, Bernard came to Dublin only a month after his father's death. He unpacked his bags at Dublin because his step-brother believed our structured daily routine and individual attention would do him good. His dorm parent that freshman year is convinced that Bernard was both relieved and "freed" by the regularity and stability of a routine to begin absorbing whatever he could from nearly everyone at Dublin. In a safe place peopled with teachers and peers who cared for the person Bernard was eager to become, he drank deeply from the fountain.

He now remembers how miserable he was during his first month at Dublin, missing his mother and feeling guilty for having left her at home alone. Understandably, Bernard needed—and received—a psychologist's counseling to help him grieve and unburden himself of guilt. From his first morning of classes in October, when his senior roommate taught him how to tie his tie and showed him to his first class, to his last day at Dublin, Bernard learned what it felt like to be accepted into a community. It was a road, he is now convinced, that made all the difference.

His first friends came in the dorm. His roommate helped him belong by being "cool" to him in the commons area when others weren't sure who he was. Then the dorm parent capitalized on a common interest in science fiction, and from there they built a friendship—one that Bernard knew also was with one of those "authority figures." With friendships solidifying in his second semester, his grades began to climb followed closely by his self-confidence. Forming another close friendship with the downhill ski coach helped him stand even taller, and enjoying cycling in the spring semester helped him feel the year had ended in triumph.

During his sophomore year, it was yet another close friendship with the younger of two dorm parents —with hours of board games and ultimate frisbee— that Bernard believes helped him make the honor roll and a better and better impression on those around him. "We had fun together and he trusted me. Totally. I considered him a kind of older proctor: a friend, but someone who was also responsible for making sure I got enough sleep and completed my homework," Bernard says now of that relationship. "It's always a two-way street. If you open up to adults and are willing to form a friendship, they will treat you like an equal. But you have to accept them—with both their roles." Bernard's advice to current students is simple: "Talk. Try to get to know your dorm parents. They are there to watch out for you." An "attitude," Bernard points out, is the worst thing to bring with you to Dublin unless you are intent on just passing through.

More than any other student his first dorm parent or I have seen at Dublin in the past five years, Bernard learned who he wanted to become through the diverse and numerous relationships he cultivated over four years of living in close proximity with both teenagers and adults.

As his sophomore and senior English teacher, I can testify to a dramatic improvement in his writing over the years. In addition, his hard work as both a cyclist and runner paid rich dividends by his senior year. As a junior he shared the honor of winning the School's coveted "spirit of Dublin" award with a classmate who also never stopped looking for ways to contribute to school life. He began his senior year as a proctor in one dorm then was the obvious choice to transfer when trouble brewed in another dorm.

Having grown independent of our school community, Bernard left Dublin for a selective college. It doesn't surprise anyone at Dublin that Bernard is a sophomore RA in a dorm of 45 freshmen. He "connected" with and learned something from everyone at Dublin. His freshman dorm parent agrees that it was Bernard's active participation in so many activities and relationships that helped form the free-standing young man who still, to this day, listens to your every word with a gee-whiz look in his eyes.

Bernard grew up and out of boarding school like many of our students who learn, from familiarity with adults, not to be awed by anyone—including presidential candidates stumping during a primary—but to be honest with everyone. Especially themselves.

New Beginnings

Teenagers at Dublin have to work hard in the classroom to make honors grades, and they have to work hard—like all teenagers —to learn the difference between knowledge and wisdom. At small schools like Dublin, however, they have new ''parents'' who help them feel part of a community. When a faculty member dies or an unborn faculty child is diagnosed with Downs Syndrome, news travels quickly and they begin to participate more actively, some sooner and faster than others, in their own lives by witnessing others—adults and teenagers—becoming intimately familiar with each other's pain. And when the diagnosis proves wrong, they learn in a place where it feels safe to feel affection that they have more in common with their new parents than they thought. From that kind of sharing they are just a step away from realizing what many sons and daughters acknowledge in their 20s or 30s: that their own parents are, like their own dorm parents, human beings also subjected to the vicissitudes of life and who, like them, often make mistakes. They are not, therefore, Mr. and Mrs. Darth Vader.

New beginnings need not depend on such emotional earthquakes, though. The tremors of any adolescent's daily life, often thinly disguised aftershocks lingering from earlier unresolved conflicts, are much easier to detect when being sensitive to them is one of the top priorities. You've got to give the edge to boarding-school parents at schools like Dublin simply because they are not ''successful'' without being good with someone else's children. There are more of them parenting at small schools—more than there can possibly be at home—and they speak in voices not already too familiar. Community, after all, is just another kind of family whose Latin derivatives literally refer to those who ''serve'' or ''give'' together.

But let's not forget the family rules, rules, rules: the lights- out rule, the smoking rule, the riding permission rule, and the unwritten don't-lie-to-your-dorm-parent rule. Throw in a ''bust,'' suspension or expulsion and we no longer have Eldorado's happy land where kings are kissed on both cheeks and children play marbles with a fortune in jewels. Instead we have something like a world where you drive on the right side of the road and can't bounce checks (unless you are voted into office). Teachers no longer paddle students, but in boarding schools everywhere they survive only if they develop that healthy suspicion of teenagers who will likely grow up to get speeding tickets and even bounce a check or two. "Small school" also means the kind of familiarity that breeds a good-humored vigilance and make secrets nearly impossible to keep.

But Eldorado's insulated existence—and its capacity to erase individuality in its seemingly rich citizens—is not, actually, what makes anyone happy. No good boarding school wants its student body sheltered from a life with consequences. On the contrary, its house rules are meant to reflect its own view of how best to raise a family. Although small schools in particular cannot afford to believe they have all the right answers (like any family), they are obligated to continue defining the limits within which their teenagers can experiment.

The Dublin Priority

What distinguishes our small boarding school's around-the-clock education is, therefore, that it necessarily emphasizes negotiation over confrontation in relationships as well as discipline. It will emphasize the process by which relationships are respected as covenants made between teenage students and the institution whose teachers coach and live with them *in loco parentis*. Many boarding school teachers have their own young families, too, but, at Dublin, families and students eat together—shoulder to shoulder—at both lunch and dinner, formal and informal, nearly every day of the week. Those teachers are also advisors to three, four, five, or as many as six students each year, and, because of the weekly "official" advisor meetings and all the other informal contact and advisee group trips off campus, it's not uncommon for students to remain with the same advisor for two or three years. Neglect is not much of a problem at Dublin.

Most important, though, is how living and learning in such close proximity demonstrates that education is more than just good grades, good scores and trophies. It is a lifestyle. Questions nagging an imbecile narrator in *The Sound and the Fury*, a student in a calculus class or a teenager sobbing at one o'clock in the morning signify much more than "nothing." Those questions become the stones on which they will step, skip, and slip their way in and out of personal and professional relationships for the rest of their lives.

A school such as Dublin, then, is a place about understanding what it takes to cultivate relationships of mutual respect and support (without any place to hide when the ride gets bumpy). There are all kinds of places to hide at larger schools. We are more interested in our students asking some of the right questions than we are in them having the right answers or getting into the right college. We are more about collaboration than competition, and we are even now considering a curriculum of design-challenges which teams of students would solve.

It is not that we are uninterested in colleges, good SAT scores, and winning games or races. Our daily all-school meetings are often punctuated with applause recognizing students and faculty for their accomplishments and distinctions. April brings good news from the colleges at Dublin, too. It is that we believe the boarding school you choose will recommend a lifestyle that may differ significantly from others because of an important difference in perspective and proportions. Certainly there are teachers at all schools—boarding and day—who help teenagers feel accepted and nurtured because those teachers also teach through relationships. But there's an unmistakable difference between a school with a few such teachers and a school which fosters in all its teachers this kind of perspective. Just ask our students who have come from other boarding schools, who in some cases have turned down a "top" school for a few years at Dublin.

No boarding school disposes of parents, but some try harder than others to work with them in helping their children understand how they can become the unique individuals they want so much to become. Any teacher will agree that self-esteem and achievement form the self-perpetuating cycle of growth that carries each of us closer to that goal, so the more that parents at home and parents at school can conspire in motivating teenage students to participate in their own education, the more likely it is that those students will achieve success—the kind that opens doors—as well as believe in themselves. Not all Dublin students need all the attention we pay them, but those who do not seem to understand quickly enough what helping us help others can do both for them and their schoolmates. All the way around, that spells community, and at Dublin that community is good for us all.

To the Parents at Home

Mister Rogers is right. Each of us has special gifts, and teachers *in loco parentis* must, if they hope to teach through relationships, believe in the uniqueness of each student and have this in mind as they live with them. But teaching in and out of the classroom through relationships proves to me that Mister Rogers is wrong, too.

Everyone is like everyone else when it comes to how we bleed and what we need. Teenagers who step, skip, and slip can suffer the most from feeling isolated by their differences. Learning in small classes and small dorms how much we are all alike, then, is at least as important as learning how we are different (or smarter or faster) because it teaches us the empathy and patience we need to belong more happily with others.

Certainly parents and their children need to understand, first, that not all teachers at any school, small or large, are always good at what they do—or that they even agree completely on their school's mission and how to achieve it. They may not even belong at their schools and, like other professionals, will move from job to job looking for the right match. An ongoing discussion at Dublin keeps us, thankfully, communicating with each other frequently so that we are continuously refining both our goals and methods.

But parents—and increasingly their children—also need to ask good questions when they choose a boarding school because they are choosing those ideas and values which will earnestly try to mold teenagers to a lifestyle, one way or the other. Because living with more or less familiarity, "pretending" or prestige will likely determine how those adolescents form their adult relationships. Parents and their teenagers need to choose carefully.

How do we live and work with other people? The SATs don't answer that question, but Mister Rogers certainly does—and so does Dublin. For students and faculty at larger schools, "going off to school" means that many kids and their parents lose countless opportunities to experience and resolve conflict face to face. In fact, those teenagers often experience a distancing from their parents which results directly from their leaving home and missing out on both the conflict and the intimacy with their own parents.

Many parents of students at Dublin come to understand that our teaching "style" means that their kids (our students) learn better how to live and work with other people. It's an education that softens one kid's tone of voice during calls home or teaches another how to keep the world from spinning so fast at the same time as it teaches math or history or chemistry or art. A Dublin education is always about learning how people are more important than subjects.

5

The Hidden Curriculum in the Dorm

by Burch Ford, Dean of Students
Milton Academy
Milton, Massachusetts

In a boarding school, the dorm is home for the students: not just where they sleep and keep their belongings, but also where they can retreat, relax, have fun, feel safe and feel cared about. Dorms are also like home where lots of the dreams and dilemmas of growing up get played out, for better or for worse.

The different levels of adolescent development (intellectual, physical, social, spiritual, emotional) all lurch along approximately simultaneously and, though it may not be so obvious, there is a curriculum in the dormitories to address that development. The adults in the dorms are teachers with a curriculum more subtle than the course plans of the classroom or the game plans of athletics. The dorm curriculum is based on the relationships between dorm faculty and the students living with them.

Students' intellectual progress—their study skills, their homework, their planning and organization of time to do short- and long-term assignments—needs attention in the dorms. Dorm faculty look after kids' physical development, their eating, sleeping, exercising, and health. Like parents, adults in the dorms need to tend to their students' recreational activities, like smoking, drinking, partying. The curriculum means helping students with their relationships (parents, teachers, friends, same sex, opposite sex, sexual behavior) and keeping them company while they sift through and sort out their own ethics and social conscience, the choices they have and the decisions they make.

The most effective learning takes place in the context of a relationship. That relationship is most crucial when the learning has to do with personal growth, emotional and spiritual. The dorm curriculum involves teaching youngsters about healthy relationships which include both affection and accountability; the

45

first part's easy, the second is not. It includes teaching boys and girls to be on good terms with themselves first and then with others, to learn to be responsible for themselves and to be responsible to others. In discussing one of the women in her studies, Carol Gilligan (*In a Different Voice*) speaks of a young woman's assumption that "morality stems from attachment." The dorm curriculum includes the creation of an ethical ethos in and through which youngsters learn about right and wrong in relation to themselves and others.

The dorm curriculum also includes teaching the values on which all the school rules are based: safety and health, integrity and trustworthiness, kindness and respect. In one of his short stories, "The Christian Roommate," John Updike says that someone with no convictions has no powers of resistance. A task of the dorm faculty is helping kids strengthen their own convictions and develop the courage to know what to resist and what to pursue in their own best interests, as well as that of others around them.

The role of the adult that youngsters in a dorm call forth is that of a logician, an administrator and, essentially, that of a parent. It's a simple concept, but anyone who has children, and most who don't, recognize what a complicated task parenthood is with a couple of children, not to mention anywhere from 10 to 50. Yet parenthood is a choice that most make, not unlike the choice adults have made to work and live with young people in boarding schools. Perhaps it's because we believe that there's no better investment of adult energy and wisdom, for short or long term returns, than in the education and healthy growth of our young. Christa McAuliffe said it best: "I touch the future. I teach."

As the boundaries in our culture have become more and more blurred about right and wrong, and as the boundaries between adolescence and adulthood continue to be blurred, the need of young people for adult protection, guidance, clarity and instruction is great. And as it is increasingly clear that we live in a culture that has no real interest in the safe and healthy passage of our children through adolescence, only as consumers and potential sources of profit, the caring and careful presence of adults in the lives of young people now is more important than ever.

Besides the physical energy it takes to run a dorm (I found one of the hardest things about being in a dorm was not being able to go to bed when I wanted to), the emotional energy required is enormous. A principal drain on the emotional reserves is having to tolerate and deal with a fair amount of conflict arising most often around terms of the contract a student makes in coming to live in a dorm (curfew, cleanliness, kindness, cooperation, communication) or issues of rules (dishonesty, drinking, lying, stealing). As more and more adults in our culture feel less and less confident about their ability to make clear demands and expectations (other than for high achievement) and to set clear, consistent limits on children's behavior, or to know what are appropriate examples to set for young people, the more important are the school values and expectations and the more parents look to schools to provide the social and ethical structure that they themselves may not feel competent to provide for their children.

A challenge of parenthood and of running a dorm is being the heavy, holding kids to what (despite their protestations) is really in their best interests. Most kids respect the adult who can risk the anger and hostility of students to do what he or she thinks is right. Kids realize how hard it is for adults who are essentially warm and caring to set and maintain firm limits. One of the measures of adulthood, learning to be one's own authority, is something that all kids aspire to, but they need adults to model for them the courage and conviction that takes. In the dorm where adolescent impulses and anxieties get played out, there's a powerful need among many students to know that things motivated by those impulses and anxieties will not get out of control (like cruelty, drinking, not eating, sexual pressure, vomiting, stealing) and there's real relief (though not necessarily for the students involved in the particular behavior, at least not at that time) when limits are made clear.

An example of this was an incident involving a rowing coach several years ago. At a practice, his boats were approaching a bridge which they had to go under when they noticed there were some boys on the bridge dropping large pieces of logs into the water. The coach took his launch to shore and ran to the bridge; the boys hopped on their bikes and started to ride away. The coach, realizing he couldn't catch them, called to them to stop and to come back. They hesitated. One yelled, "You're not my father." Another said, "We don't have to." The coach responded, "Yes, you do." They reluctantly came back to the bridge. The coach explained to them the danger they were putting the rowers and the boats in. Some understanding seemed to have been reached; the town boys apologized and went on their way. The practice resumed with no mention of what happened. Later on, the young rowers told their friends how great the coach had been. They had clearly been frightened by the falling logs, excited by their coach's chase and confrontation with the other boys and, ultimately, impressed and relieved that their coach's action had protected them from harm, had stopped the destructive behavior of the others, and had brought order to a situation that threatened to get out of control. I suspect the town boys were also grateful and relieved on some level. They were prevented from harming someone and some valuable property and, hence, were spared the consequences (conscience, parents, school) of their intended behavior had it gone unchecked, and may have learned something in the process.

The same relief at adult intervention is felt when the situation is one of verbal hazing, physical bullying or some form of cruelty, food fights, fist fights, suicidal behavior, chemical dependence, eating disorders, stealing. Kids recognize and respect the courage it takes to intervene when ignorance, indifference or abdication would be the easier, and perhaps more familiar, position to take. They don't necessarily tell adults though, just as the rowers never told the coach how impressed they were; he learned it from a colleague who overheard the boys talking about him with admiration.

Confrontation is protection, something we all owe others we care about. By intervention and/or confrontation, I don't mean taking an adversarial position, but rather a position of recognition, acknowledgement and care that leads to a new level of self-awareness and understanding. Adolescents, like many adults, don't recognize and identify their feelings right away, and when they do, may not acknowledge them for some time, if ever. The rewards of working with adolescents have to come in part from oneself and from other adults. Fritz Perls said that a parent in need can't feed. In order for adults working and living with young people to be able to sustain the level of commitment which young people need, adults need to be nourished and sustained by other adults.

In teaching youngsters how to get along with themselves and each other, a dorm head is consciously or unconsciously doing some ethical education, teaching responsibility for oneself and responsibility to others. To live successfully in a dorm, students need to learn that what they do has implications for those around them and that they are responsible for the consequences of their own actions and behaviors, both intent and effect, the good things where credit is due and the not-so-good things where more needs to be learned. If a student does something that elicits a disciplinary response from the dorm staff, that's a learning opportunity for the student. But it takes energy and courage on the part of the adult to allow that to happen. The dorm staff can teach the student that it was the student's choice of behavior that elicited the negative consequences; it was not the teacher's choice to respond. Sometimes the adults are as confused as the student and feel guilty for responding to the student's impulsive or thoughtless behavior.

There's also important learning and teaching that takes place when a student does something well, when he or she comes down on the right side of a struggle. There's an assumption among us, I think, that if we've done something well or right, we know it; and if we do something that needs improvement, we owe it to each other to say something. In fact, we're often shooting from the hip and need to know it when we've hit our mark. If this is true for adults, how much more must it be for kids; the ones who seem to intuitively handle their lives well are often the ones we attend to least. Also, understanding the process of healthy, positive decisions can be just as instructive as learning from one's mistakes.

The narcissism that's a normal part of adolescence has to be outgrown for adulthood to be achieved, and the dorm is a place where kids can learn the limitations of their egotism, where they can learn some alternative actions and perspectives to move beyond their self-centeredness, where they can learn about the power and comfort of community. From the teaching and example of dorm faculty, young people can learn to be more clear about what may enhance themselves and their community and can move closer to healthy, constructive choices and decisions.

To do the job in the dorm well, to manage all the pieces of the curriculum, takes enormous amounts of physical and emotional stamina and that of which none of us has enough: time. A while ago, Doonesbury ran a series of interviews with Dr. Dan Ascher, the Tastemaker to the Mellow. In one segment, Dr. Dan was discussing the concept of quality time in his new book, *The Mellow Parent or Sharing Your Space with Dependents*. Dr. Dan was asked exactly what quality time was. He responded that it was time each day that had to be devoted to a child; it didn't have to be much, ten minutes was usually enough. But it couldn't be spent watching television or something; quality time had to be spent addressing the child's needs. The interviewer asked what if one of the child's need was more time. Dr. Dan responded that that was quantity time and that he wasn't talking about the problem child here!!! Appealing as it might have been to busy parents, that was an idea whose time (such a pun) will never really come. Relationships of any substance can only develop over time, with trust and, ultimately, talk. Dorm faculty know that lesson well; part of their role is to teach that lesson to their students.

A dorm faculty can't really replicate parents, nor the dorm a family; they can approximate both. Like parenthood, the cost to the dorm teachers is considerable, but the value to the student inestimable. Keeping expectations realistic (e.g. dorm staff can't be there for 10 or 50 kids the way they could for a few; some students have struggles that the best dorm staff in the world couldn't resolve alone and perhaps couldn't even with the added resources of other faculty and health services; running a dorm well requires that staff have support and appreciation from some source other than students) can help keep the curriculum fresh and in focus and preserve some adult energy, not just for sharing in students' struggles and victories, but also their own.

To paraphrase Freud, youngsters in dorms need to learn to find the balance of love, work and play. That's what dorm faculty have to teach. That's the stuff of the dorm curriculum.

6

"Operation Blackout" and Other Reflections on Dorm Life

by John T. Conner
Groton School
Groton, Massachusetts

By early October, 1978, I had survived my first full month at Oakwood School in Poughkeepsie, New York, where I was teaching Spanish and running the ground floor of a boys dormitory. This was my first year as a teacher and my first experience in a private school; I had little idea what to expect. I was on duty four nights a week and every other weekend. One of my rare Friday evenings off, I had invited a fellow first-year teacher, Dale, to my apartment for dinner. If she and I were to have any privacy, she would have to sneak in. I had already learned that when my students knew I was in—door open, door closed—I would be constantly interrupted.

Dale arrived a little before 6 p.m. when most of the boys were at dinner. We immediately began "Operation Blackout," an elaborate scheme to convince the boys we weren't there. Before dinner I had parked my car across campus near the gymnasium; it was now time to hang heavy woolen blankets over the windows— no cars outside, no lights visible inside. Next, we put pillows on the floor in front of the door leading to the dormitory hallway and pressed masking tape to cover the small cracks on the top and sides of the door. We unplugged the telephone, lit some candles, and began to cook dinner, speaking in whispers.

Soon the trouble began. As boys returned from dinner we could hear them speaking in the hallway. The walls were so thin we heard nearly every word. "Do you think John is in?" said one of them. (Oakwood, proud of its informality, put us instantly on a first-name basis.) "Let's find out," said another as he knocked. Dale and I stayed dead quiet. We looked at each other, looked at the door, and didn't move an inch. The knocking continued. "Hello, anyone home?" We remained frozen and, as I stood in the dark, I realized I was a prisoner in my own home.

The boys moved away, and we continued to prepare dinner. I placed a juicy steak in a frying pan in my "kitchenette." Kitchenettes are often provided to dormitory heads to make them feel they have all the comforts of home. My mini-refrigerator could barely hold two six-packs and a dozen eggs. Its "freezer" could make one mini-tray of ice, and my two-burner electric stove was one step up from a hot plate; I often felt as if I was living back in my college dormitory. Soon the smell of onions and meat wafted through the air. "Do you think they'll be able to smell that? asked Dale. "No way," I said. "How could the smell get through the door?"

Five minutes later my question was answered as the knocking started again. "John . . . Hey, John . . . anyone home?" We remained silent. A few seconds passed and then a loud banging made us think the door was about to be knocked down. A boy was pounding it with a hammer. "Open up, John. We know you're in there," cried the boy. "Boy does that smell good . . . can we have some?" I rose to my feet in a fury, kicked away the pillows and flung open the door, ripping the masking tape. Standing sheepishly in the hall was a pack of five boys. Smiles came to their faces when they saw Dale, the candlelit room, and the beautifully set table. One boy nervously said: "Here's that hammer I borrowed yesterday. Th-th-th-anks a lot." Another boy asked if I had change for a dollar, while another asked what the Spanish homework was. I couldn't help smiling as I listened to these brilliantly concocted excuses to see what their dormitory head was up to on a Friday evening.

I am finishing my ninth year living in a dormitory. Since 1981 I have worked at the Groton School in Massachusetts. I came eager to run a dormitory, but had to wait three years for one to become available. At Groton, dormitories are named after the dormitory head. Hence, I have been running Conner's Dormitory for eight years. I do what many teachers at boarding school do: teach a full load of courses, coach two varsity sports, run a dormitory of twenty-one boys, proctor study hall, serve on numerous committees and perform other assorted duties. While the hours can seem overwhelming at times, the combination of duties is very appealing. Living in the dormitory has given me an opportunity to get to know young people in a very personal way. As a dormitory head, I have accepted the considerable responsibility to protect and nurture these young people who live away from their parents. I would like to share some of the wonderful experiences I have had, mention some misgivings, and finally offer some suggestions for school administrators and fellow dormitory heads.

What's Great

At its best, a dormitory acts like a large, if somewhat unusual, family. Students and faculty are all dependent on one another and see each other most times of the day and night. Being around a motivated, intelligent, and, for the most part, polite group of young people invigorates me. I have enjoyed the hours spent discussing school issues and news of my students' lives. I like having the chance to help students with homework, to congratulate them on their achievements, and to try to make their stay happier. I feel I am able to get to know students in a different, more intense, way than I am able to in my classroom or on the athletic field. Simply put, running a dormitory can be fun. It is particularly gratifying to have students stay in my dormitory for more than one year; it is exciting to watch these boys grow up.

I can remember many fun and zany events in the dormitory: being carried to the showers for a dowsing when I announced my engagement in 1988 . . . a tradition had been established by the boys for "showering" any person who was officially going out with a girl (traditions at boarding schools can develop in a matter of weeks); inviting the boys into our apartment for weekly "feeds" (a Groton term for late night snacks; among the favorites are: pizza, roast beef sandwiches, brownies—it is best if half a bag of chocolate chips is added to the recipe—ice cream sundaes, and cold cereal) which also feature lively discussions, joking around, and occasional musical or audio-visual entertainment (a group of boys last year could perfectly lip-sync Michael Jackson's "Man in the Mirror," while some boys this year can do a perfect cover for Wilson Phillips "Hold On"; one year we made a dormitory video production entitled "How to Study for Final Examinations" in which each boy was asked to offer his dormmates special, and not necessarily very serious, exam-taking tips); heading out for a sledding trip to a nearby mountain; going to a bowling alley for a Sunday afternoon bowl-a-thon; having an all-dormitory slumber party in my living room with my air-conditioner on full blast one unusually hot spring evening; taking part in an outing last May for the spring formal called "The 'Za-dyssey" when boys in my dormitory and their dates were chauffeured by limousine to the Groton House of Pizza for a sumptuous dinner complete with pizza, live music and belly dancing; "McShuttling" the boys to McDonalds during examination week; cooking hamburgers outdoors for a picnic; and having push-up contests in my apartment.

Looking back, I can now laugh about what happened one snowy evening after we had made a fire in the common room fireplace. I was in my apartment and every so often I heard what sounded like a small explosion. I went out and saw all the boys seated around the fire. I commented that the wood in the hearth must be very dry since it was crackling so loudly. I learned after graduation that once I was back in my apartment out of earshot, the boys had erupted with laughter. It turns out some had been tossing small firecrackers into the fire. Old, gullible, Señor Conner himself had provided a plausible alibi.

Potential Problems

During my early years working in boarding schools, I had some real shocks. Before coming to Groton, I was at one school where there was a good deal of drug use, in general and in my dormitory, to which I was oblivious. One day in the winter, the headmaster summoned the dormitory heads into his office. Wearing a fire chief hat to add some levity to a very serious meeting, he announced there were reports that LSD was being used on campus. Consequently, he had decided there would be a room search. A student could turn in any contraband before the search began without penalty; if the subsequent room search turned up any drugs or alcohol, the student would face disciplinary penalties. As I went from room to room with a dean, I was amazed at what my students turned in. By the time it was over we had collected a large garbage bag full of empty beer cans, half-filled alcohol bottles, marijuana, and numerous water pipes, a.k.a. "bongs." No LSD was discovered, but the search opened my eyes to the rampant rule-breaking. Later that year, students admitted to me that these room searches had been quite amateurish. One student showed me how he could easily remove the platter from his turntable; earlier in the year, including the day of the search, he had hidden here many plastic bags full of marijuana. In thinking back on these events, I can't help but feel that we adults had not been providing enough supervision and help for our students. A room search is certainly a drastic measure, but one that may be needed in certain circumstances. When issues of student safety collide with student privacy, I think that schools should err on the side of safety. This incident helped me realize the many problems inherent in residential schools.

First and foremost, there is the problem of establishing enough adult presence in the dormitory. With 20 students to supervise and a full schedule of events starting with chapel early in the morning and ending, at least in the winter, with evening sports practices, I often feel I do not have enough time to spend with students. There are evenings, too, when I want to spend time with my family or prepare for classes. For the most part, dormitories at boarding schools are unsupervised between 11 p.m. and 8 a.m.. During my teaching career, I have *never* been directly instructed to wander through the dormitory during these hours. Many boarding students know when they will be free from adult view. While I have been told I should "always feel free" to go through the dormitory at any time, that statement is quite different from a directive to do so. Occasionally, on my own initiative, I walk through the dormitory late at night to be sure that all is quiet and settled.

An adult presence ensures that rules are followed and gives kids the feeling of protection and guidance. Dormitory heads have so many children to look out for that they don't always feel confident they are providing the necessary care. I often wonder if my students are getting enough sleep, getting to breakfast, finishing their homework, keeping their rooms neat, doing their work program, observing curfew, following drug and alcohol rules, being kind to their roommates and dormmates, brushing their teeth before bed, and feeling secure and comfortable. Given that it is not easy for adolescents to live away from their parents, do I feel I am doing all I can to make this experience a healthy and positive one? Am I spending enough time with each student? How would I feel if all these children were my own? Although these questions are not easy to answer, they should be considered by dormitory faculty regularly. The more time that a faculty member is able to spend with students in the dormitory, the better the chance that students may be influenced positively. By developing a good relationship with students, a faculty member is in a position to be able to address many important issues directly with students.

Suggestions

I would like to offer the following ideas to school officials and fellow dormitory heads:

All faculty should share dormitory duty

All faculty who work at boarding schools should share in the running of the dormitories. One of the strengths of Groton is that *all* faculty share this responsibility. Dormitory faculty cover three nights a week, and non-dormitory faculty, called affiliates, substitute three nights a week. Affiliates run study hall, do check-in, supervise work program, and are available to stay overnight when needed. Each member of the faculty is also assigned to Saturday evening duty once a month. I know that there are a number of schools where the dormitory heads alone shoulder all the evening responsibilities. Not only does this exacerbate the differences between dormitory heads and others, but it may also result in an unhealthy school ethos. Resentment directed towards non-dormitory faculty can become intense. Dormitory heads need some evenings off; affiliates need to understand, first hand, the dynamics of dormitory life; and students enjoy getting to know all their teachers in more familial surroundings. I have been lucky to have one affiliate who guards my dormitory door like Cerberus, the three-headed dog of Hades, allowing no one to interrupt me except in the case of emergency. Affiliates provide a system for protecting the privacy of a dormitory head on a night off. The small dinner party I described at the beginning of the chapter would have been a lot smoother had an affiliate been on duty.

Dorm rules should be posted

All rules related to school life should be posted on a dormitory bulletin board. Rules should be explicitly stated and repeated frequently. Schools can open themselves to unnecessary difficulties by certain vagueness. For instance, a discipline case involving alcohol became muddled recently because rules had not been written down explicitly. Some of the key questions were: Was being in the presence of a person who was drinking alcohol equivalent to drinking alcohol oneself? What does probation mean? There was considerable turmoil and anguish felt by many of my colleagues as well as by many students when the decision that was approved seemed to contradict what many of us had thought were the operating rules. In my opinion it does a young person a great disservice to operate with murky, loopholed rules. However well-meaning they may be, it is a dangerous sort of "compassion" that gives students "a break" when they have clearly violated the spirit and intention of a rule. Students need to know there will be a predictable response to certain behaviors. This year many of the rules have been clarified; they have been posted in the dormitories, and there have been far fewer disciplinary cases than usual. I believe these three facts are related.

Bedtimes should be established

Adolescents need plenty of sleep; when they do not get enough sleep there are deleterious effects on mood and performance ("Patterns of Sleep and Sleepiness in Adolescents" by Mary Carskadon *Pediatrician* Volume 17, Number 1, 1990). Responsible parents monitor their children's sleep carefully. Boarding schools should do the same. While Groton has bedtimes for its eighth and ninth graders, we currently do not have a bedtime for any of our tenth, eleventh, or twelfth graders. There are too many students who do not get enough sleep. While a case can be made that seniors are old enough to set their own hours, schools should have a lights-out policy (possibly 11 p.m. for sophomores and juniors). Students could petition for special "late night" privileges on occasion.

Compensation

Teachers who run dormitories should receive financial compensation. Schools should also make the living quarters in the dormitory as pleasant as possible. Groton's dormitory housing is superb; many of the apartments, in fact, are larger and more attractive than some of the school houses. Running a dormitory is a time-consuming responsibility. School administrators should be aware of this when assigning teaching loads, athletic coaching, committee work, extra study hall duties, etc. While some inequities are inevitable, school administrators should work very hard to distribute the workload fairly.

The headmaster, assistant headmaster, and deans should be very visible

A healthy school needs to make both students and teachers feel that what they are doing is noticed. A school administration should help establish an adult presence in the dormitory. My recommendation is that a dean *and* either the headmaster or assistant head make at least *two* visits per week to each dormitory. If the dormitory head isn't there at the time, the administrator should make a point after every visit to leave a note or report personally what was observed. These visits can last for as little as a few minutes; I am absolutely convinced that student morale is lifted when they know the head honchos check to be sure a dormitory is neat, see that there is quiet in the evening with studying going on, and notice a special event in the dormitory. There have been times during my career when I was not sure if a dean had visited my dormitory during an entire term. Dormitory heads should not be made to feel isolated or left on their own to supervise children outside of classes. They need to know that rules are being followed consistently around campus; it is not fair to require one's own students to make their beds daily when other dormitory heads do not require the same. It is up to the school administrators to be sure consistency occurs. I become annoyed whenever I hear a faculty member forwarding an argument that suggests that a "student's room is his castle"—that is, inside his own room a student should basically be able to do what he wants. In my opinion, this type of operating principle has no place in boarding schools. Simply put, a student is under the care and supervision of the faculty of a school. The responsibility of safety and nurturing belongs to the school. Expectations and rules are in force at all times; there can be no "free zones" where one is immune from watch or accountability.

Inspection sheets

About five years ago I began to leave little sheets of paper for each student with comments about the room's cleanliness. A few boys began to post these little slips on their walls. That same year, one of the Deans came around frequently to my dormitory. After his visits, he would leave a type-written report in my mailbox describing each room. I was amazed to discover the interest my boys took in this written report. They asked me to read it to them and delighted in receiving good reviews. I think they also did not mind bad reviews. The key idea was that they were happy that someone was noticing what they did. By giving some sort of formal recognition to non-academic areas of school life, dormitory faculty may help to influence students positively. Three years ago I decided to post daily inspection reports on the dormitory bulletin board. I now do these inspections every day without exception, Monday through Saturday. On Sunday evening at 8 there is also a grand formal room inspection when I check for careful vacuuming, dusting, and empty garbage cans. On a daily basis I check for made beds and general order. Each day I also include a "word of the day" —a new vocabulary word I think will be helpful to a student's working vocabulary. I write out a definition, then use the word in a sentence. At least twice per term there is a vocabulary quiz given at check-in. A dormitory average over 90 percent earns a special feed. I have never had a group score below that level. Below are some sample inspection sheets from last fall:

CONNER'S DORMITORY
ROOM INSPECTION
DATE: THURSDAY, OCTOBER 31

Happy Halloween

Room 301:   I would like to see a better effort here tomorrow . . . the vacuum could be used, clothes and papers picked up . . . overall quite uninspiring today.

Room 302:   This room proves positively that there is life after death. What a difference from yesterday! Your RESTRICTION is over.

Room 303:   Solid as a rock. DORM BEST

Room 304:   No mirage today, just abject mediocrity. Does a bold new wave await me tomorrow? I (and you) hope so.

Room 305:   Excellent effort marred only by contraband material (a dining hall cup) conspicuously atop a desk. You came quite close to a dorm best today.

Room 306:   I would like the desks and top of bureaus cleaned off by tomorrow. There is too much paper, empty bottles, and miscellaneous material here; it destroys what would be an amazing view from the doorway.

Room 307:   Solid, professional effort. DORM BEST

NOTE: THERE WERE A FEW MERITORIOUS PERFORMANCES TODAY, BUT OVERALL I WAS NOT SWEPT AWAY BY YOUR EFFORTS. I HOPE FOR MUCH BETTER TOMORROW!

Word of the Day: "cryptic" an adjective meaning "mysterious, puzzling, enigmatic" . . . In a sentence: "When I was walking through the cemetery, I heard a number of cryptic comments being made by the ghouls, ghosts, and goblins who had just escaped from their crypts." (This sentence contains a play on words . . . .I hope that you chuckled; if not, please re-read.)

CONNER'S DORMITORY
ROOM INSPECTION
DATE: MONDAY, NOVEMBER 4

Room 301:   Overall very good; the beds could be made a little neater.

Room 302:   The bed with the red cover should be more neatly made; I am also considering reporting you to the *American Society for the Prevention of Cruelty to Plants*; the big plant by the couch is crying for water.

Room 303:   It's not often that I am able to offer suggestions, but there was a gum wrapper on the floor, the bureau was not perfect, and a Hobart door was open. Overall, the look is still good.

Room 304:   DORM BEST. DORM BEST. DORM BEST. DORM BEST. A new day has dawned in Unit 14. Phoenix-like, Room 304 has risen from the ashes to take the premiere spot of cleanliness today. I was astounded by the careful attention you gave to every detail. The progressively larger bottles on the bureau certainly proved to be an eye-catcher. Great effort.

Room 305:   Close Hobart door, put away pair of pants from the Killer Chair, straighten desk; otherwise quite good.

Room 306:   Excellent job today; some picking up under the bed nearest the door would make it perfect. Runner-up, DORM BEST

Room 307:   I can't tell for sure whether or not the vacuum has been used within the last 24 hours; it looks like a small vacuuming could be therapeutic. Overall, good.

Room 308:   Middling (as in "fair to middling"). I'd like to see some greater attention to small (and big) details by tomorrow.

Word of the Day: "prandial" an adjective meaning "of a meal, especially." In a sentence: "The post-prandial activity in the dormitory last night (after the last cinnamon rolls were devoured) was work program."

PLEASE NOTE: TONIGHT THERE WILL BE A FEED AT CHECK-IN TO CELEBRATE THE SUPERB CHAPEL TALK GIVEN THIS MORNING BY ONE OF OUR DISTINGUISHED PREFECTS.

I spend approximately 40 minutes each day doing an inspection and writing up reviews. Although I have many busy days, I regard this responsibility as sacrosanct. These sheets provide extra daily direct contact between my students and me.

Handshaking

Check-in at night should take place in a central area, even if it is only in a hallway. The responsibility for check-in must rest with the students. Dormitory heads should not be reduced to playing "Hide and Go Seek," searching room to room (including checking bathroom stalls) to be certain that a student is in the building. Students should check in, shake hands with the dormitory head, and stay there until everyone is present. This time is a good one for important announcements and group fellowship.

Feeds and Special Events

The school should try to supply each dormitory with a small budget that will allow a weekly evening snack. At Groton we are given approximately 15 to 20 dollars a week. My wife and I are then able to have the boys into our apartment for a snack. We may light a fire or put on special music to provide a relaxed setting. My students always look forward to coming into our home; the small change of scenery from time to time is eagerly awaited. I also try to encourage the boys to think up some events to do together such as a picnic, movie, outing to go sledding, or a trip to a local restaurant. Although each dormitory head will feel comfortable doing different things, I think that the willingness of a dormitory head to organize such events is important. These are the types of activities that are remembered for many years by students. It is a wonderful way for students and faculty to socialize together.

Evaluation/Feedback

Good administrators should make it their business to know what is going on in the dormitories. They should solicit topics of discussions for regular meetings of dormitory heads. They should ask us to get together occasionally on our own without deans or other administrators. In that meeting dormitory heads could be asked to put together a list of suggestions for what further support could be offered them by the administration. If dormitory heads ever report frustrations, administrators must be certain to deal expeditiously with these issues. There is nothing worse than waiting for a response that doesn't come. When there are good things that happen in the dormitories, there should be public mention of them. If a dormitory is especially neat, if a special event happens, someone must make it his or her business to take notice.

For example, when faculty go to great lengths to be sure their dormitories are left clean in June at the end of the school year, they should be commended. Many of my fellow colleagues feel that usually the shortcomings get noticed rather than the good things. In a similar vein, because dormitory people are often those who are in the position to become involved in disciplinary cases (most of school rule-breaking occurs during non-academic hours), dormitory heads often spend a lot of time and painful effort enforcing the rules. It is, therefore, important that administrators make a point of telling dormitory faculty personally that they are glad we are doing our job. Often dormitory heads feel that administrators will react to reports of rule-breaking or of other problems like the Wicked Witch of the West from the Broadway musical *The Wiz* who sang the rousing tune: "Don't Nobody Bring Me No Bad News." I think this feeling would subside if deans and heads of schools frequently said things like: "I can't thank you enough for doing your job well. The fact that you caught Roger last week breaking a rule may help him to turn his life around here. It also will set a good example to the rest of the school. Thank you for the hours you spent on this case and that you spend in the dormitory; I realize there is a lot of talk from students who criticize teachers for being 'police agents' or 'out to bust.' Just know that in my book you are doing your job well. I, and the school, are grateful to you."

Be creative, energetic, and fun

Finally, a dormitory is largely dependent upon the energy and creativity of the dormitory head. Adolescents respond very well to attention, humor, and loving care. If the time ever comes when being on dormitory duty consistently feels like a chore, it may be time to get out. Administrators must work hard to make housing available outside the dormitory for people who have put in many years. What happens in school dormitories is too important to be left to teachers who feel burned out.

As I head off to Spain next fall with my family on sabbatical, one of the things I will miss most about Groton will be running my dormitory. I will be sad not to be able to work with my fourth and fifth formers (sophomores and juniors) who might have decided to stay in Conner's dormitory next year. It will also be strange to have the dormitory "renamed." I wonder if the alumni of my dormitory are doing well wherever they are living.

The promise of a healthy experience in a residential school is made possible only by the determination of school administrators and faculty members. There are few areas of a school that would not be helped by improving the quality of life in the dormitory. At its best, a dormitory is a wonderful place to be. The experiences that children can have living together under the watchful eye of a caring faculty member can be very valuable. I hope that an increased discussion of residential issues will offer a new vitality and feeling of common purpose to the faculty who are in charge of this crucial area of boarding school life.

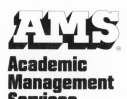

7

Of Risks And Riches

by Joy Sawyer Mulligan
Director of Admission & Financial Aid
The Thacher School
Ojai, California

"Why on earth did the Admission Committee accept this kid?"
It is a thought held in wonder or puzzlement or even anger, at least once in every faculty member's tenure at a given school. Sometimes it is spoken aloud, in a faculty meeting or at a teachers-only lunch table, or half-muttered in a hallway between classes. That the question is in teachers' consciousness or on their lips suggests the necessity of some kind of dialogue about students whom we might term admission "risks" and about the school cultures in which they might be at risk. Before beginning, though, lets recognize that defining risks is something akin to nailing jello to a wall. It's more than a little messy, certainly difficult— but what a wonderful texture! And what a challenge for us all as educators!

Consider this as the launch pad: Together, as teachers, administrators and admission staff, set aside some prime faculty meeting time to ask a tough but utterly essential question: "what basic skills and attitudes do young people need to function well—successfully and happily—in our school?" (Query students, alumni/ae, parents too. Any overlap on your lists? If not, you have some work to do in that area.) Some examples of "ways in" to answer that question are: Is yours a school that places a high premium on individual responsibility early on in a student's tenure there, or are youngsters' hands held fast and firm throughout most of their time with you? With what sort of achievement records have most of your already-proven students entered: mostly A's? A's and B's? C's and D's? The whole gamut? To what extent are learning differences, disabilities and deficiencies appreciated and accommodated? Which, if either, is valued in your school: community or autonomy? What level of maturity do you expect of students entering at the bottom rung?

These questions-to-answer-THE-question—only a few among myriad others possible—encompass an entire landscape of academic, social, emotional and developmental issues. The answers to them, taken collectively, also represent the special and often specialized cultures of our schools, the idiosyncratic environments into which we bring young hearts and minds.

Once you have determined the particular landscape of your school, you will begin to see its boundaries—boundaries that differ and vary widely from school to school and that are sometimes in flux even within an institution, as leadership and staff change. Here then enters the question of risk, for it is at these edges that risk—for the student and the school—lie. When by virtue of an admission decision, we expose (but not necessarily subject) a student to any kind of damage or loss—of self-esteem, of "place" or identity, of a sense of self as valued and unique—we perforce pose a similar hazard to our school. Educational consultant and former admission director Frank Stephenson calls this "threatening the center," the larger area in which students fit our schools' norm in all the aspects noted above. Having to invest too much more than our "usual" care in a boy or girl (however that "usual" is defined) is to dally with uncertain danger—uncertain because we can never know exactly what repercussions will ensue, or for whom, or how severe they might be. Some possibilities are: the student may become the target for resentment among other students who feel, by contrast, neglected; the faculty advisor and classroom teacher may feel unfairly burdened by academic, emotional or social needs which they did not anticipate or for which they are not trained or prepared; parents may wonder why their child was admitted in the first place if everyone involved wasn't willing to go that extra distance. In short, disillusionment and dissatisfaction ultimately spell disruption for the school community on a small or large scale. While these consequences or others like them do not inevitably follow every risk admission, their potential lurks. We all—admission officers and teaching faculty—must be aware of their shadowy presence.

From both the admission perspective and that of the faculty, knowing exactly the nature, extent and strength of your school's support net is crucial to understanding the extent to which risk is a factor in admitting and then embracing any given student and, we would hope, to avoiding the disruption of the "center" alluded to above. The various strands of the net's warp and woof, the tightness or looseness of its weave—these determine the extent to which a student is or is not truly a risk or at risk. Classroom teachers, faculty advisors, prefects or proctors, peer counselors, dormitory heads or staff, coaches, a school counselor, big brothers and sisters, learning specialists, a study skills teacher: the defining and interweaving of these roles (and others), then the establishing of a clear and useable system of communication among the people in the roles, administrators and parents, creates your school's particular net. Admission directors must bear the responsibility not merely of knowing their school's support systems theoretically, but of having had enough intimate contact with them (by being or having been an advisor, teacher or the like) to be able to represent them to prospective students and their parents with authority and anecdotal specificity. Faculty members and administrators must be clear about and comfortable with the various support roles they are asked to assume in their schools.

All this is not to say we should never take a leap of faith on individual students. Most of our schools cannot afford not to, from both a practical, economical point of view and a perhaps higher, more philosophical one. A carefully, sensitively, thoughtfully considered decision to admit a student who just might bring with him or her certain but, we hope, temporary shortcomings of skill or character (or even more irrevocable deficiencies of aptitude) could at once yield an exquisitely rich educational experience for all concerned. (Keeping a file on those success stories prompts hope to spring eternal among admission folks and such students' teachers.) And the pure diversity that comes along in the suitcases of a girl who just spent her 7th and 8th grade years living on a sailboat taking even a middling good correspondence course or a boy from a one-room schoolhouse town in Montana: that is a spice, a piquancy without which our communities would be flavorless and drab.

In taking these leaps, however, we must not act on blind faith but must—for everyone's and our institutions' sakes—find roots in some reality. And the grounding reality that our collective experience tells us to seek in a youngster is the element of passion. If a boy or girl, in other ways marginally qualified for your school, demonstrates a keenness, a proven commitment over the course of time to something—almost anything—he or she will have a source of strength and comfort and identity when all else (algebra, soccer, a roommate) seems impossibly difficult—but then, only if your school can nurture that something. (A rabid and accomplished figure skater will not be well served by a boarding school in southern California.) Entrance exam scores in the lower reaches, mediocre achievement in school, lukewarm academic recommendations from former teachers: for an admission committee, these should recede in importance when a youngster can claim a niche of excellence, a place wherein his or her sense of self has already nestled, secure and unshakable, before he arrives at your school's doorstep.

Such risk students, attended to with care and understanding, often do find acceptance and success in our schools; they triumph in ways we might never have imagined as we considered them for admission. But which ones do not? The answer, individual for each of our schools, can be found in a relatively simple, long-term "risk audit" of sorts: the admission director and dean of students should keep close track, year by year, both of those students about whom the admission committee had reservations of any kind (academic, social, developmental, emotional) and those who come to "threaten the center" without having had any red, or even pink flags in the files as candidates. In looking at these students, do you see a pattern on their transcripts or in their teachers' comments or advisor reports, similarities in their difficulties or the challenges they present to teachers and staff? Surely some of the students considered risky admits throw that term back at us; we gladly make the catch and in doing so perhaps refine our definition of those boundaries alluded to above. But those who begin as risks and remain so, and those who become harmful to themselves and to the community as they live with us, can give us inestimably important information about ourselves as schools and about the extent of institutional tolerance of such students.

By systematically tracking these students' successes and failures, both as individuals and as a group, we better serve prospective candidates and their families. We know with far greater authority and certainty what works and what does not, how far to the fringes we can venture in an acceptance and still provide at least a modicum of safety for the student and the school. We have an inventory of the skills and qualities held by those students functioning ably in our school; a sense of how tightly plaited our school's nets of faculty and staff support are; an eye for a candidate's unmitigated ardor for excellence in an activity; the knowledge of our responsibilities in this system and to a marginal student. Yet even with all these tasks accomplished, the original "Why on earth?" question still raises its voice. Why indeed? Because of a final wild card: the single, most desirable, most suitable candidate, whom an admission committee might vote "Most Likely To Succeed," comes into an environment—your school's particularized culture—that for some unpredictable, often untraceable, reason is simply wrong for that boy or girl. In this sense, as one of my colleagues in admission says, "They're all risks, every one of them."

Not a very reassuring thought, granted. But wild cards are sufficiently rare, both in poker and—if we all are doing our jobs—in schools. While uncertainties are, paradoxically, a fixed part of working with adolescents, those we call risks, both in admission and throughout their enrollment, can be surer bets.

Recommendations: Forging an Admission-Faculty Team on Risks

Directors of admission should consider:

- Having classroom teachers represented in a sensible rotation on the Admission Committee or in some other meaningful advisory capacity to raise awareness of faculty concerns for incoming students at risk.
- Informing faculty who will be a particular risk admit's support net of that student's specific weaknesses, as well as talents and strengths that may help pull him or her through; discussing the family background with these teachers to whatever degree is appropriate; meeting as a group as time permits to assess the youngster's progress and growth.
- Joining with the dean of students (or corresponding administrator) to track risk enrollees, then sharing resulting observations with faculty as part of an ongoing discussion on student-school "match."
- Noticing, supporting, encouraging and applauding the work of advisors, teachers, counselors and others in specific ways: in notes of appreciation, aloud in faculty meetings when appropriate, among others.
- Devoting one faculty meeting annually to a discussion of admission policies

and practices. In one of these, you might conduct an all-faculty mock admission committee meeting, utilizing the files (names changed) of students recently graduated. Some surprises await!

Faculty members should consider:

- Joining any volunteer efforts offered by the admission office (actual committee work, other in-house ambassador programs, informal open houses) to understand better the intricacies and challenges of the admission effort and to be a positive part of it.
- Welcoming any opportunity (on a pathway, in a hall, at a lunch table, at the door of your classroom) to have contact with candidates and their parents to gain a sense of the kinds of families investigating your school.
- Keeping the admission director or other officers informed of academic or behavioral difficulties you have with new students especially, not with a "Why on earth?" approach, but in the spirit of systematic communication about the whole issue of risks.
- Accepting the inevitability of teaching, advising and coaching risk candidates.

8

The Evolution of an Anti-drug, Anti-alcohol Program

by James H. Wilson, Chairperson,
Dormitory Life Committee
The Loomis Chaffee School
Windsor, Connecticut

It was sometime after the Saturday night check-in (11:30). Having accounted for everyone, the person on duty, Brenda, was casually wandering around the dorm, making sure that everyone seemed settled. She heard some laughter and noise in one room, knocked, and after what seemed like a prolonged pause, was invited to enter. Three boys were sitting around listening to music, yet each of them looked unusually tense. Brenda was sure she smelled beer, so sure that she said, "I think I smell beer in this room. Have any of you been drinking?" The boys quickly denied knowledge of any beer being in the room—making it sound as if they hardly knew what beer was! But Brenda, still uncomfortable, felt sure she really did smell something. She told the boys not to leave the room, that she wanted to get her dorm head for a "second opinion." As Brenda left the room, she was thinking to herself that they might really have to conduct a room search, which, according to school policy, should be conducted with a dean or dorm head and always with the resident of the room present. No one ever looks forward to conducting a room search. She headed off to find the dorm head, two flights down and at the other end of the building, leaving the door to the student's room open.

Meanwhile the boys snatched the open beers and additional cans which were under the bed, took them to the janitor's closet, and placed all the beers in a secret hiding place behind some ceiling panels which were easily removed and replaced to conceal such illegal substances. They used some mouthwash an↵

aired out the room before Brenda and her dorm head returned. Obviously the
boys continued to deny any consumption of beer and, predictably, none was
found when conducting the search.

Though this scenario probably sounds familiar to many boarding school people, it was for us the enactment of a role play among boarding school faculty
about 15 years ago. Then, as we were trying to better understand student use of
drugs and alcohol and to define and coordinate our responses, we met about once
a month, sometimes to do role plays of this nature. We laugh now about that
session; although we felt it was entirely appropriate for Brenda to question the
boys directly and follow up with an investigation—that in itself was a somewhat
bold approach at that time in response to such a suspicion—we laugh at her/our
naivete at leaving the boys alone in the room while she went to seek help. This
was part of the trial-and-error process through which the faculty at our school
came to grips with the use of drugs and alcohol on campus.

The fact that we have had, and continue to have, sessions such as these
indicates that we know ours is a drug- and alcohol-using society, and that, yes,
we are a part of that larger society. Yes, we have had to suspend and dismiss
some students for use. And yes, we are uneasy about the use of these substances
by our students and particularly about what sometimes seems, among older prep
school and college kids, to be almost a frantic devotion to weekend parties. This
concerns us greatly, and it does not take a genius to know from whom young
people have learned such behavior. It is one of those ongoing problems that will
never be "solved."

But our present students confirm over and over, that one does not have to use
drugs/alcohol to be "cool"; most students on campus do not party and there is
little or no peer pressure to drink or smoke pot during the school term. Just this
fall, in three different admission interviews, parents asked me about the drug and
alcohol situation at LC. In each case they said that their student tour guide (who
had no previous prompting on this issue) said (to quote one of them), "Yes,
students do use drugs and alcohol sometimes, just as they do everywhere. But at
Loomis you are not pressured to do so—you are accepted if you choose not to.
There is plenty of peer pressure not to use drugs." And another student who is
presently a junior and has been at Loomis Chaffee for three years summarized
this view nicely by saying, "At Loomis the drugs don't find you; you find the
drugs." That is to say, if you wish, yes, a student can find drugs in the greater
Hartford area and bring them onto campus. But there are few instances in which
students are pressuring their peers to drink or smoke pot.

Why does this attitude prevail among the students, and how have the attitudes
and school policies evolved in the past 15 years to a point where we feel we have
a pretty good grip on what is a problem of ongoing concern?

Twelve years ago we were pretty naive. As a dorm resident for 32 years, I
know that I and my dorm staff were ambushed by the use of drugs in the
mid-70s. We didn't understand them and didn't know how to respond. We gave

a lot of mixed messages by our failure to react and probably encouraged more kids to continue smoking pot than we realized. I can recall numerous cases in which all the signs of drug use were there and I failed to respond.

The first thing we really did, in 1979, under the leadership of a small faculty committee headed by the director of counseling, was form a faculty Drug and Alcohol Committee (DAC) which invited some "experts" to tell us what was going on. This included several day-long workshops plus monthly meetings for faculty, especially those living in the dorms. Some were with doctors and active drug counselors; some were with drug-enforcement agents who actually showed us what we were dealing with; some were with psychologists. Perhaps the biggest impact came from leaders of a group called "Freedom from Chemical Dependency" who met with us, shared their personal stories of addiction, denial, confrontation, and the process of recovery, and guided us about how to respond. Since then—for 12 years now—this group comes for five days each fall to meet with all our sophomores, as well as faculty and school leaders. During that week, each sophomore is excused from four or five class periods to meet with about a dozen classmates and a member of the FCD staff. During these sessions, FCD staff provide hard information about various drugs (including alcohol), tell their own personal stories, and respond to student questions; it is not uncommon for a student to express some concern about his or her own drug use or, more often, about how to help a friend or relative who has a drug problem.

In addition, we have a large counseling staff which includes several full time people and nearly a dozen other adults who also teach, live in dorms, coach, and have a special interest in working with young people on a formal counseling basis. The director of counseling runs an orientation program each fall for new faculty about how to respond to student use of drugs and alcohol. It can be extremely nerve-wracking to confront a student, especially for a younger faculty member who may be only five or six years older. During the early 80s, an Alateen program was established here on campus; this group continues to operate and serve our students today. So, step one was education and conversation about what previously had been an issue we pretty much avoided in hopes that it would "go away." And we are constantly seeking to "update" ourselves with new information and new insights into adolescent behavior.

The next thing we explored was how to respond. We found this to be a far greater challenge than just acquiring the information. Now we had to put our beliefs on the line and learn to confront students in a forceful yet fair way. This part of our training involved doing a lot of role plays and then having our faculty group-critique what had transpired. One such role play is described at the beginning of this article. These were not easy at first; we were reluctant to actually confront students unless the "smoking gun" was present, for it takes a lot of self-confidence and courage to "bust" a student. Not surprisingly, most of us dreaded such confrontations and feared that in challenging a student about his or her use of drugs, we might in fact be wrong. Every adult in the community has had to overcome the fear of being "disliked" and called a "narc" for challenging a suspected user or turning an offender into the deans. Word travels quickly on our island! (LC is often referred to as "The Island" because at flood time in the spring, we are surrounded by water from the local rivers.)

We have a community in which there exists a good deal of trust between faculty and students, and we did not want this to be jeopardized by hasty accusations. Yet, we knew we could not look the other way and we were convinced the community, as well as individual students in the community, would be happier and better served if we were absolutely clear, in our words and actions, about our beliefs and the rules.

We did role plays on walking in on students actually drinking; we did them on the situation when a student checks into the dorm or comes to class looking a little "out of it"; we explored how to confront a student whose grades were slipping and who was losing interest in his sports or other activities. We discussed and played out the situations where a faculty member has heard a rumor that Johnny or Susie has been drinking on campus. These sessions lead to numerous conversations and debates about the meaning of "confidentiality," something we take seriously at Loomis Chaffee, especially in counseling situations. How does one respond, for example, when he or she learns, perhaps from an advisee, in confidence, that the student has a real drinking problem? Can we still maintain the confidence?

The more we got into it, the more we recognized that we would, on occasion, have to confront and help young people already addicted; in some cases the issue was far more than simply a matter of discipline. We worked these things through in a lot of meetings, discussions, and role plays. Sometimes we included Student Council members or dorm prefects in our discussions. And all these conversations and role plays have, more than anything, served as a valuable support system for faculty. One does not feel alone when confronted with a situation involving a student who may be using drugs and alcohol. We have a mandate, from each other as well as from the headmaster and the deans, to act on these issues, and we have many colleagues with whom we can share our concerns and anxieties about how to respond. Over the years it has proven a great source of comfort for faculty to feel such support.

In addition to the integration of student leaders into our meetings, several faculty members organized an adolescent peer counseling and support group that actively brought in speakers to talk with students and conduct sessions, usually without adults present, about drug-related problems and how peers might help each other. More than a few students who felt alone as non-users or felt uncomfortable with their own use valued the opportunity to talk about these issues in an open student forum. In a few instances, a student with a dependency was brought, by his or her peers, into fruitful counseling before he or she was caught and possibly dismissed.

Twenty years ago we probably would not have responded at all to drug or alcohol use unless it was a blatant violation of our rules; today we do not hesitate to confront, in a respectful manner, a student whom we suspect. A teacher may do this if a student looks "blown" in class, or an advisor may do the same if there is a sudden change in grades or conduct. Or a dean or coach may question a student. We have learned how to do this in a manner that still respects the student and his or her innocence until proven guilty. Every time there is a double message: first, the obvious reminder is, "Watch out! We are watching! You could get yourself into real trouble with the school if you are using drugs or continue to do so!" And the more subtle and probably more important message is: *We care about you.*

My very strong sense is that students want to have the rules clearly defined and expect them to be enforced. They lose respect for us if we do not confront rule-breakers. Many students think we know more than we do and sometimes wonder why we don't do anything. I recall one such incident a few years ago. I was on duty one Saturday night and at around 11:30 students came to check in. I was tutoring a student so as each dorm resident appeared, I told him just to come over to the desk where I was seated and check his name off. Very simple. The next day several of the prefects told me that a couple of kids in the dorm were really nervous because they thought I wanted each person to get close to me so I could check his breath. They worried all night that I would come to their room at any moment to bust them! I guess, in retrospect, I was the only one who didn't know what was going on! But I also learned from the experience, thanks to my dorm prefects. And this incident was the basis for a role play at our next DAC meeting, and we discussed at length whether or not I should have confronted the students the following day after the prefects had identified the suspicious characters. The fact that the offending students thought I was checking on them probably had a positive effect on all. But the fact that I did not respond, especially since they thought I knew what was going on, may have served to encourage even more drinking. Crazy!

It became obvious that it was essential we all, especially the 35-40 dorm resident faculty, have a unified position about the use of drugs and alcohol, knew what to look for, and prepared a coordinated set of responses. Too often in the past our faculty were not clear on just what the school rules were, let alone having a clear sense of how to enforce them. We put together a handbook for faculty on how to respond to a whole series of situations —from slight suspicion (a student simply acting strangely at a dorm check-in for example) to the situation in which a faculty member walks into a room where a joint is being shared or a beer is being drunk. These guidelines included concrete suggestions on how to proceed, when it was appropriate to call a dean, or when one must involve the health center or a counselor. We always stressed the importance of not turning one's back and of following up with the student, be it a day or a week later, be it once or many times during the year. Many faculty have found that after a confrontation—these do not happen often—it is much easier for the adult and the student to talk about drug and alcohol use.

We have worked hard as a faculty to define our rules on drug and alcohol use. Any student caught using or in possession of any kind of illegal drugs or alcohol is suspended for four days; when the deans feel that sending a student home would place an unreasonable financial burden on the parents, the student will remain on campus and do 15 hours of work for the school; during those four days, the student may not participate in classes, athletics or other school activities. Although we are not always entirely comfortable with the idea of having a student miss academics for this long, we do believe that the time spent at home with one's parents is valuable, and because most suspensions include all or part of a weekend, most suspended students miss only two, sometimes three, class days. Upon returning to school, and after the offender and his/her parents meet with the dean, he or she is required to meet with the school's psychiatrist (at the parent's expense) for an evaluation and referral to either a therapist or a school counselor. Often the psychiatrist will ask to meet with the parents as well. We feel it is important to invest the parents in the process, if only by having them pay for these sessions.

In addition to these steps, the student is placed on what we call a Level II disciplinary standing. This means that if there is another violation of any major school rule (not only rules about possession or use of drugs and alcohol but also about cheating, stealing, leaving campus without permission, hazing, destruction of the property of others, violation of the parietal rules and so forth), that student comes before the Disciplinary Committee with a recommendation for dismissal. Unless there are quite extraordinary circumstances, the student is dismissed. Exceptions occur if the student has had an exceptionally good record for a long period of time between offenses. Fifteen years ago we tended to be a bit softhearted and thus frequently found reason not to dismiss a student after his or her second offense; the result was confusion in the minds of the students and, as mentioned, a willingness to take more risks.

Originally we tended to view student use of drugs and alcohol as a disciplinary issue. But, as we began to dig more deeply and came to better understand drug use and the reasons for it, especially among young people, we recognized the problem is also a counseling issue. In most cases it is the violation of a school rule that brings the problem to our attention. Once the punishment has been served, however, we meet the student head on with every opportunity for counseling to help him come to grips with the problem, be it simply a teenage mistake in judgment or some degree of dependency. Frequently the follow-up counseling reveals alcohol use and addiction in the family.

Our director of counseling recalls the case of a young man who was busted early in the boy's junior year; the boy received counseling for nearly two years. He went to Alateen, but not regularly; the boy's father was an active alcoholic, his mother an enabler. Despite the fact that the counselor and the boy worked well together, the boy continued to have problems with alcohol during his first two years in college. Only as a college junior did he really get things straightened out, and now he is a regular member of AA. This is just one of many cases in which we realize we might not make a difference now, but have planted seeds that may grow later. That's the faith all educators must have.

We learned early on that we could not save every dependent kid. There were two students in particular to whom several faculty advisors and counselors devoted an enormous amount of time, monitoring their lives, taking them to AA, and providing them with extensive counseling and support. It didn't work. We learned that it was too much strain on our resources, that we cannot follow what one might call "the hospital model"; both of those youngsters needed 24-hour service by professionals. Despite our strong urge to serve, even "save" a youngster, all committed teachers and counselors learn that sometimes the efforts take too much away from others in the school and that the dependent student(s) has to be referred to those with more time and expertise. That's OK!

There have been times when we have felt it would be simpler, possibly a stronger deterrent, if we said, "One offense and you are out." But we have resisted taking what we consider to be somewhat of a simplistic stand, largely because we are dealing with young people, who will make mistakes, and we feel that within reasonable bounds, we can help a student who has erred. Most students who break a major school rule once do not do so again. There are enough "success stories," situations in which we feel we have really helped a student come to grips with peer pressure and even some chemical dependency, that we like our "second chance" philosophy and practice. Conversations with students make it clear that by allowing them a second chance, they do not see the school as giving a double message or lacking in resolve. My own impression, from talks with teachers and deans at schools at which first-time offenders are dismissed, is that because of the severity of the punishment, faculty and student leaders are sometimes reluctant to turn kids in and rarely, of course, is the student ever able to get help from people who have come to know and care about him.

Every situation seems to be different and few are simple applications of the rule book. But we believe that step one is to make sure the rules are clear in the minds of the faculty and students. This was not always the case. Sometimes in the past faculty would know a student was using marijuana and talk with him, thus unintentionally allowing him a kind of "safe haven" which was interpreted by the student as allowing him to smoke. This tacit endorsement frequently encouraged that student (and his or her friends) to take more chances, often with harmful consequences; frequently, when, as adults, we do not actively take a stand against some behavior, young people assume we approve of those actions. In the early 80s, I became aware that a student in my dorm was smoking pot quite regularly. After several conversations, he admitted it to me and I came to believe that, through my counseling, I was "saving" him. In fact, just the opposite occurred; he came to believe that as long as he talked with me, he could continue to smoke on campus, that somehow continuing to talk about it made it OK. After all, I knew and I hadn't busted him! Eventually he was busted and, a month or so later, expelled. In the process, numerous "clean" students in the dorm became increasingly cynical about the school rules and lost respect for me and the dorm faculty in general who seemed to be approving and enabling this student to continue his habits. In retrospect it would have been much better to have forced the boy to face the disciplinary process, then get him the kind of counseling and therapy he needed. It was not until the young man had completed college that he got his social and emotional life in order. Other faculty have learned from similar experiences.

Besides trying to enforce the school rules and provide counseling for those who have broken them or are in some way drug dependent, our educational effort has been somewhat broader in scope. Our message—in small groups with sophomores, in dorm meetings, at all-school convocations, and in many one-on-one conversations with students and school leaders—is that using drugs, including alcohol, in order to relate socially is actually detrimental to one's social growth. Rather than going through the normal adjustment straight, they "cheat" by using drugs to relax and to socialize; it's a little like using a steroid to get strong.

We continue in the 90s to discuss these many situations and our proper response. Some of this discussion takes place among the whole faculty, some among deans and dorm faculty, much of it among the seven or eight faculty affiliated with each dorm. As in all aspects of teaching, we have to guard against getting lulled into expecting immediate results. We also sometimes run the risk of simply getting tired of fighting the battle. It is not a task, like building a house, which at some point is complete. The combined educational-disciplinary-counseling effort starts anew each year with new student leaders, 200 new students, and a handful of new faculty.

In the area of drug and alcohol counseling (and discipline is often an integral part of the counseling process), great expectations are a sure-fire means to frustration and disappointment. Busting and counseling a youngster may not yield tangible results until he has graduated, and frequently we may never know the actual results and whether or not we helped. One must believe in the rules and the reasons for them and care enough for the young person's welfare to persevere. Our concern is not just with the user. As head of a freshman-sophomore dorm I am particularly concerned about defending those youngsters—a very large majority—who are serious about their schoolwork, their sports and their personal growth and consequently do not feel the need to drink or use drugs because they want to live by the rules. They need and deserve our support!

It may be that the most important reason students do not feel pressure to use drug and alcohol here at LC is that the student leaders have taken a strong and consistent stand against such use on campus. Their position is partly the result of who they are, what they value, their own sense of self worth, and our careful selection process. In choosing students to be our dormitory prefects, we are very clear about not tolerating any compromising when it comes to living by the major rules. The prefects are chosen by the faculty dormitory heads from a large number of candidates only after a series of interviews and careful discussion involving all the dorm faculty. The process of selecting prefects is very deliberate. Any student prefect caught violating a major school rule is dismissed from his or her position of responsibility immediately.

It should also be noted that in our training of dormitory prefects, while we do not require them to "turn in" any known violators of our drugs and alcohol rules, we do expect them to do something positive; and we outline for them a whole list of possible responses including speaking with the offender, warning him or her that if the behavior continues faculty will be informed, going to the dorm head or dean, or seeking out a counselor. Obviously it is crucial that there be open communication and trust between the prefects and the dormitory head.

Student prefects receive training prior to assuming their very important dorm positions. All of the prefects attend an overnight retreat on a weekend in May, prior to the year they assume their duties, and have several training sessions during the fall. At these sessions, old prefects share their experiences, the new prefects role play situations that will likely occur in the dorm, and they develop a sense of unity and mutual trust. Over Labor Day weekend I take my six junior prefects to Vermont for a few days of camping, hiking, bonding, and trust-building; while we discuss many of the problems they are likely to encounter, including students using drugs and alcohol, and ways in which they might respond, the most important part of this time spent together is to build a common sense of trust and mission. Throughout the year the prefects meet about once a month as a group, sometimes to hear outside speakers, sometimes to discuss boarding school issues with the dorm heads, and sometimes among themselves to consider their own responsibilities and evaluate how they are carrying out those prefect duties. Most important are the weekly meetings each group of prefects has with the dorm head. Sometimes these meetings are driven by an agenda of dorm issues and persons who need some special attention; at other times, the prefects and dorm head (and often the two other dorm resident faculty) gather to socialize and talk generally about the dorm and perhaps plan some dorm event or activity.

Most of these student leaders have succeeded in school and achieved positions of leadership without relying on drugs and alcohol, and in the all-prefect training sessions, at which these issues are discussed, a lot of mutual reinforcement takes place. These are kids who know from their own experience that they do not have to break rules and rely on drugs and alcohol in order to do well, feel good, or be well-liked. Most are convinced that substance use in school can only interfere with their achievement.

Besides understanding that being a leader requires one to live by all the rules, our student leaders have had excellent role models in their younger years here.

In my dorm, for example, I presently have six junior prefects who have been truly outstanding role models, having learned from the standard set by the individuals who preceded them. There is no magic formula for having strong leaders, but once this kind of leadership is in place, it is often self-perpetuating. It is also essential to have adults who are willing and able to take the time to help young people develop leadership qualities.

A wonderful example of how our system can work took place early this past fall. Two junior prefects noted that a new sophomore was using drugs and warned him that if he continued, they would have to report their strong suspicions to me. A few weeks later the prefects learned this same student was still using drugs. They then reported the boy to me. We confronted him and he quickly admitted he had been drinking at a dance; consequently he faced the disciplinary system and was placed on Level II. Because he lived a long distance from school, he had an "on-campus suspension" and received counseling. About a month later, however, the several prefects came to me again and reported they had strong suspicions the boy was still smoking pot, though they had not actually caught him in the act. We organized an intervention which involved bringing the boy before two prefects, the director of counseling, and myself. The outcome was that he admitted he could not really stop on his own and went on to receive professional counseling. In this case, the line between actually being caught and being taken to the dean on the one hand, and going to intense counseling on the other may seem a bit fuzzy. But because the boy had not actually been caught the second time, it was entirely appropriate to bypass the disciplinary system. Had he been "caught" a second time, he'd have been subject to dismissal, and he knows that will happen if he is caught drinking or smoking pot again. The boy seems to be doing fine.

This story demonstrates that there are student leaders who care enough about the school rules and about an individual to report this offense in the first instance, and get him help when it appeared he could not reform on his own. This is really a story about caring! It was a gutsy thing to do, but these student leaders never doubted for a minute that it was the right thing. As expected, the prefects took a little "heat" from some upperclass acquaintances, but they accepted this as part of the price to pay in getting younger kids off on the right foot and living by our rules. As the dorm head, I was not totally surprised by their actions, yet was impressed by their very strong sense of commitment and concern for this younger dorm resident. A very clear message was given to the other 34 student underclassmen in the dorm as well as to sophomores contemplating applying to be prefects the following year. Not only has the particular boy been greatly helped, but the dorm is a happier place. The students know where they stand, and those who are trying to live by the rules feel supported by the student prefects as well as by the faculty. To be sure, it would have been more difficult for a senior prefect to turn in one of his classmates on his senior corridor, but the fact is our leaders do care and are willing to take a firm stand on these very sensitive issues. What terrific on-the-job leadership training for these 17-year-old prefects!

Yes, student leaders have broken major rules, but not often, and in each case he or she is removed from the leadership position and is subject to the normal school penalties. Obviously it is essential that we hold our school leaders to the highest possible standards. Junior prefects who have broken a major school rule are allowed to apply for prefectship the following year.

Unlike in most of the situations described in *Casualties of Privilege*, faculty at Loomis Chaffee are present nearly all the time. We are a school of over 700 students. Half the student body goes home at night. With over 80 percent of the faculty living on campus, the student-faculty ratio in the boarding school is about 4:1 or 5:1. Faculty make their presence felt in the dorms. Three faculty actually live in each dorm, and there has evolved a powerful "open-door" tradition. At LC students know they can visit faculty in their apartments and homes for extra help or to talk about almost anything. As faculty we do sacrifice some privacy, but we accept this as part of our mission. Dorm residents do the weekend duty, which means being in or around the dorm most of the day Saturday, all of Saturday evening until at least 1 a.m. and all of Sunday. We have made this a top priority partly because we believe that the quality of community life depends on our presence and partly because our headmaster and deans continue to impress upon all boarding faculty how important it is to help create a comfortable and supportive living environment for our students. Teenagers need interested adults to be present for support and as role models.

This kind of attention and support is possible because of the student-faculty ratio. Besides dorm duties, the 80 percent of faculty living on campus assume other boarding duties including monitoring evening study hall, the computer room, and the art center on school nights and on weekends, chaperoning dances and on-campus gatherings or driving vans to local events. As a dorm resident, I have official dormitory duties every three weekends. Rather than suffering burn-out, my colleagues and I have the time and energy to informally visit with advisees and generally "hang out" in the dorm; we can be supportive or just be available; we can organize some activity or trip. In this way, it does not seem as though we are "checking up on them"; rather it is entirely natural for adults to be around. If any school desires thorough dormitory supervision, it must define "duties" in such a way that those involved are not overwhelmed by excessive responsibilities within or outside the dorm. For most faculty, classroom teaching comes first; for many, coaching takes a good deal of additional time. Unless the headmaster makes proper provision, dorms will be run by burned-out faculty, and this simply does not and will not work!

In addition to the three faculty members who live in each dorm, four or five others, who live in campus housing and who have advisees in the dorm, each come in one night a week to do duty from 7 until around 11. Sometimes on weekends there is a planned and organized dorm event—an "open house," a movie and snacks, a skating party or a bike trip or hike. More often the faculty person on duty simply visits with kids in the dorm, in the social room, on the corridor, and in student rooms. We also gather by dorm three nights a week at a "family style" dinner which provides one more avenue for informal and honest communication between the dorm students and the seven or eight affiliated faculty. As a result, much of the easy interaction between students and faculty happens "naturally"; it seems to have always been this way. Students expect us to be around and they become accustomed to having easy access to the dorm faculty in particular, be it to get a light bulb, watch TV, seek help with homework, or just visit and chat.

Yes, surely there are times after 1 or 2 in the morning when faculty are not moving around and when kids certainly can and do drink or smoke pot in their rooms. My impression is that this occurs no more frequently than it does for those living at home. The faculty committee of dormitory heads and deans meets monthly to share concerns about dorm and campus life. Unlike some schools, where faculty disappear before or after dinner, it is a tradition at LC for faculty to be present. This is, I believe, fundamental if a school is to have a grip on the problem of drug and alcohol use.

It should also be noted that faculty set an excellent example in terms of their own use of alcohol and even smoking. Very few faculty smoke cigarettes and we have informally come to an understanding which makes us very reluctant to drink when students are around. This is not a faculty mandate, but rather an indication of how strongly we generally feel about our position as important role models.

Some observers of the school might think that having 350 day students would make our campus all the more open to drugs and alcohol, and there certainly have been instances in which day students have been "suppliers" for boarders. We have caught some, obviously missed a few. But the 50-50 boarding-day ratio actually works in our favor and for many reasons. Most important the boarding students feel they are part of a larger community than our "island." Life can be very stressful at a highly competitive college preparatory school; add the pressures all teenagers feel to be accepted and the additional pressures assumed by those in a theater production or on an interscholastic team, and you have a potential powder keg. In the adult world, we are reminded of the socially accepted response almost every time we open a magazine or watch TV: "Weekends are made for Michelob."

The fact is that our boarding students can get off campus and interact with the outside world. Sometimes they go home, often visit with day student friends, go to Hartford for a concert, movie or hockey game, with faculty members to rock climb, bike, visit a museum, or windsurf. All of this helps create good spirit and a healthy environment much more so than at schools where students are locked in for the better part of ten weeks. Parents of day students are frequently here on campus for games and other events, and many "adopt" one or two boarders as their extra sons or daughters. This means a lot to the boarding student and certainly makes his or her life more enjoyable. The day students, too, benefit greatly from being part of our national and international community in that they do not feel like "second-class" citizens which is sometimes the case at schools where the day students are a small minority.

After a tough week of homework, classes, tests, papers, games, work job, and extracurricular activities our students do need to unwind. They have a wide variety of ways in which to relax and get recharged for the coming week. Most do not feel that big-time partying is the only route; it is not the activity of choice during the school term. On one recent weekend, for example, when I was on duty, a bunch of students, boys and girls, day and boarding, went to the home of a day student for dinner, then returned to campus for our major winter dance, the Junior Informal. On the same evening, a local parent gave me a dozen tickets to the Whalers hockey game so I took a van-load to the game in Hartford. Others walked to Windsor to watch a movie ($1.59!) and grab a pizza, while a few were content to relax either in their rooms, at the snack bar, or in the social room watching a movie or the NCAA basketball tournament. Everyone was back in the dorm by 11:30, and after a snack and an hour of Saturday Night Live, most were in bed; when I went to bed at 1:15, the dorm was silent except for a couple of quiet conversations in individual rooms. During the winter, one of the favorite activities is dorm hockey and hot chocolate.

There is no "system" that will absolutely prevent student use of drugs and alcohol. There are many reasons teenagers may feel the need to use these substances, all of them learned: some do it to relieve stress, some just to "relax," some to assert their independence and adulthood, a few to rebel against authority, some for adventure, others to feel accepted, and some because they enjoy it. A few are dependent. Most of these reasons are not so very different from those that would be given by a sample group of adults. But we try to make it clear that in addition to being against our rules (and those of the state), drug and alcohol use is not an acceptable way of satisfying these social and emotional needs.

Our success has come as a result of human interaction. It is a combination of good role modeling by faculty and student leaders alike, the faculty's devotion to kids, definition and consistent enforcement of rules, a very effective and active drug and alcohol counseling program, and attentive faculty members that has helped us arrive at this point. We will never be totally satisfied which is why we continue to meet frequently to discuss these issues and redefine our responses. Like most everything in education, the dynamics of working with young people are always changing and ever challenging. One should not be involved in teaching, especially in a boarding school environment, unless one loves young people and has confidence in their potential for growth.

9

Discipline at Hyde School

by Malcolm Gauld, Head
Hyde School
Bath, Maine

As a ninth grader I read *The Headmaster*, John McPhee's biography of Frank Boyden, headmaster of Deerfield from 1902 to 1968 (not a misprint!). Perhaps I was initially fascinated by the book because I was the son of a headmaster but many of the glimpses into Boyden's life have stayed etched in my mind. I don't know which is more astounding, the fact that he held his job for 66 years or the fact that he expelled only five students during his entire tenure. When pressed on his remarkable statistic, Boyden liked to say that "a boy is more important than a rule." While we've updated Boyden to embrace co-education, as has his own school, his phrase is perhaps the operative principle in our discipline program at Hyde School.

Hyde School is an innovative school founded in the 60s, an innovative decade. Perhaps we're fortunate that our program of discipline was established during the very era in which it was expected to function. An effective discipline program is an elusive goal for all schools but can be especially difficult for older schools which must often balance old traditions with new challenges. We have come to discover that a few concepts stand the test of time:

- Honesty must be the cornerstone.
- We strive to value attitudes over infractions, ethics rather than rules, the spirit over the letter of the law.
- Students must be involved at all levels. If students want greater autonomy and increased decision-making power, they must bear the burden of even the most unpleasant facets of maintaining discipline. Schools can no longer play "cops and robbers."

A description of our experiences with the application of these principles follows.

HONESTY: Attitudes vs. infractions
BROTHER'S KEEPER
CASE STUDY: Debbie & Jim

A discussion of discipline at Hyde School must begin with our school's ethics. These concern issues of lying, cheating, stealing, sexual behavior, drugs, tobacco, alcohol and what we call Brother's Keeper. The standards pertaining to these ethics are thoroughly explained by the Dean of Students on the first night of school. Students are expected to adhere to these ethics with a positive attitude.

HONESTY: Attitudes vs. infractions

This expectation of a positive attitude constitutes much of the grey area which sometimes surfaces with teenagers in regard to rules. For example, consider a teenager who goes downtown in an attempt to buy marijuana, but is unable to locate a dealer. Has that teenager broken an ethic of the school? In a world of rules, as exists at most traditional schools, the student probably would not be penalized. (Indeed, it is doubtful that the school would ever learn of this action.) Now throw the question of attitude into the equation as we do here at Hyde. In this light, there's no question that a discipline problem is involved in this incident. As we are fond of saying, *"We do not discipline infractions at Hyde; we discipline attitudes."*

Many schools operate from what I call a discipline "menu"; infractions are listed down the left side of the page as are the entrees on a restaurant menu and the cost of each infraction is listed on the right side as are the prices. We, at Hyde, do not play that game. Here, it is entirely possible for two students to commit an infraction, such as smoking cigarettes together, and yet receive different programs of discipline because of differences in their attitudes and levels of honesty.

A veteran student will answer the following question: *"What is the most serious infraction you can commit at Hyde School?"*—with a consistent answer: "lie." While careful emphasis is placed on all the ethics, we are especially emphatic about lying. Students are expected to honor the spirit of the truth, not simply the letter of it. If I accuse Johnny of smoking Marlboros with Debbie and he thinks his denial puts him in the clear because they were, in fact, smoking Camels, Johnny is lying. Positive growth must rest on a foundation of honesty. It's no small coincidence that among Hyde's Five Words and Five Principles, three deal directly with the notion of truth. In fact, the Principle of Truth states: "Truth is our primary guide." This point is made almost incessantly to new students when they arrive at Hyde School. Before we examine specific disciplinary approaches used at Hyde School, let's take a moment to consider Brother's Keeper.

BROTHER'S KEEPER

Most of Hyde's ethics are easily understandable by anyone. The fact that we do not allow students to take drugs and that we penalize them for stealing from their peers does not surprise them; nor are students surprised to learn that cheating is not tolerated. After all, Hyde is an academic college preparatory school. The "rub" with the vast majority of Hyde students comes with the concept of Brother's Keeper. Simply put, students are expected to act upon the disciplinary infractions and attitudes of their peers. They are expected to hold each other accountable. For example, if you are not a smoker but you're walking downtown with Johnny, who lights up a cigarette, you have a responsibility to do something about it. You must tell Johnny to turn himself in to the Dean's Office and make it clear that if he doesn't, you will. If we later become aware of Johnny's smoking and it becomes clear that you knew he had smoked and that you had not acted upon it, you will be treated as if you were in the same boat as Johnny. This is a bitter pill for Hyde's students to swallow. When a young student first learns of Brother's Keeper, he or she will invariably say something like *"No way! I'm not going to 'narc' on my friends."* In most schools, a student would commit social suicide if he or she turned a classmate in for breaking the rules of the school. Not so at Hyde.

In the early stages of a student's involvement, not much time is spent explaining why Brother's Keeper is a good thing. Usually a student must experience the benefits of the concept before he or she can enforce it with a full heart. Are there benefits? The degree to which Hyde's newer students hold the concept in disdain is matched by a fierce loyalty by older, more veteran students. They understand that if, for example, three members of our basketball team are smoking, the team is simply not going to achieve what it set out to achieve as a team—its best. The players who are smoking are holding the team back. When viewed in this context, smoking is a very selfish act and benefits no one. As the Principle of Brother's Keeper formally states, "We help others achieve their best." Hyde students have learned that if they push others and others push them, the total benefit will be greater than the sum of its parts.

Part of the difficulty of the acceptance of Brother's Keeper lies in the fact that a student's initial association with the concept is usually a negative one. Either a student has committed a violation of the ethics and does not want to accept accountability for it, or one has witnessed another student committing a violation and would rather not get involved in the ugly social repercussions of turning a fellow student in. However, later on, after a student begins to perform well academically, scores a few goals out on the soccer field or sings a solo in a school production, the student realizes that he or she might never have accomplished these things without the positive peer pressure of Brother's Keeper. After these experiences the student generally regards Brother's Keeper in a positive light.

CASE STUDY: Debbie & Jim

Perhaps the best way to understand Hyde's discipline program is through a hypothetical case study. Let's follow two students through the different levels of the program. Consider a boy named Jim and his friend Debbie who are new students at Hyde School. On their first night at Hyde the Dean explains the ethics. Jim and Debbie have heard these kinds of admonitions before. Disregarding them, they then go out and smoke. An older student observes them smoking and asks them to turn themselves in to the Dean. They look at the student incredulously and say *"You've got to be kidding!?!"* They refuse to comply and the student turns Jim and Debbie in to the Dean. At that point, Jim and Debbie will separately sit down with the Dean of Students who will remind them that they made a commitment to follow the ethics of the school and having broken that commitment, need to accept some accountability. They will undoubtedly be placed on **5:30**.

Jim and Debbie will be told to meet in front of the Student Union at 5:30 on the following morning where they will be supervised by members of the Dean's Office (usually students, often those who spent a good deal of time in disciplinary activities themselves when they were younger students at Hyde) as they rake leaves, shovel snow, sweep walks, pick up litter, etc. The number of mornings that they will be expected to do this will depend completely on their attitudes. If they're on time in the morning, work reasonably hard for the hour prior to breakfast and don't lip off to their supervisors, they will likely do this for a total of three mornings. At the conclusion of their discipline, they will sit down with a group of students and faculty from the Dean's Office and discuss what they have learned from this endeavor. The commitment that they made at the interview will be re-examined and they will be expected to state in a one-page paper how they intend to follow the ethics for the remainder of the year.

I remember once when I was a young kid at the amusement park in Old Orchard Beach, Maine. Somewhere in the arcade there were a couple of benches with a sign over them which read *"Do Not Sit On These Benches."* I walked over to the bright red benches, observed the sign above them and could think of no earthly reason why someone could not sit on them. They were clearly in good order, well built, well maintained. Not only could I not think of a conceivable reason why one couldn't sit on them, I couldn't imagine why someone would go to the trouble to make a sign stating so. I then sat down on one of the benches and received an electric shock. That's the kind of kid I was. I had to see for myself. I'd say the typical Hyde student is much the same. A majority of Hyde's kids will test the ethics (to see what the fuss is all about), will serve their accountability and then will go on and do what they came here to do: learn and grow. Chances are that Jim and Debbie won't have future problems with the Dean's Office. Let's say they do.

A week later, Jim and Debbie, feeling good about the five days that they've

just spent in classes, are walking downtown. They celebrate with another cigarette, entering into a pact not to tell on the other if one is caught. Let's say that
Debbie, who is beginning to perform well in academics and sports, has a guilty
conscience over what they've done. She talks about it with the captain of the
soccer team and after this conversation decides to turn herself in. Jim is then
called in to the Dean's Office. He sticks to the pact. He doesn't tell the truth even
after he's told that Debbie has confessed to the smoking. Jim considers it a trap
of some sort and stays with his story. Even when Debbie is brought into the
room, Jim continues to lie, stating that it's his word against Debbie's (and
proving that there is little honor among thieves *and* those who violate school
ethics!) Although both students have committed the same ethical violation, we
now have a case where the two exhibit different attitudes and different levels of
respect for the truth. This calls for something stiffer than "5:30." Jim and
Debbie would then go out on what the students call **2-4.**

2-4 stands for 24-hour work crew. The student does not, in fact, work for 24
consecutive hours, but he or she is pulled out of the regular program of the
school. There will be no participation in classes, sports, nor other regularly
scheduled activities and programs. The message to the student is simple: *"Since
you have demonstrated that you do not intend to follow the Hyde program in an
honorable fashion, the school will offer you a program which is much 'easier' to
follow."* Supervised by the school's maintenance department, Jim and Debbie
will work around the grounds during the hours that other students are engaged in
the curriculum of the school. The fact that students often consider this cruel and
unusual punishment says more about our society than it does about Hyde School.
The tasks that these students are performing are those done by millions of
Americans every day in order to put bread on the table for their families. That
students will often view this as cruel and unusual punishment reminds us that
today the concept of chores is a foreign one belonging to a bygone era. In many
cases, students simply haven't been asked in the past to do many things that they
don't want to do. Thus, when they are required to do something that they truly
don't want to do, they consider it cruel and unusual. They will very well call
home and try to get their parents to bail them out of this horrible predicament.

To return to Jim and Debbie: By this point, Debbie is beginning to see Hyde
School in a more positive light. She buckles down to work for two or three days
and meets all of her obligations on time. In her Concern Meeting with the Dean's
staff it appears that she has learned something from her experience. Debbie will
be released from **2-4.** On the other hand, Jim has been showing up late, lipping
off to his supervisors, and doing all his tasks in a half-hearted manner. Chances
are good that Jim will be on **2-4** for a few more days, maybe longer.

Sometimes it can reach a point where Jim's attitude causes difficulty for his
supervisors out on the grounds. Let's assume that his insubordinate, disrespectful
conduct intensifies over time. At this point, Jim might be required to be put in
a position of what is sometimes termed "meaningless" **2-4.** In other words, he

may be expected to perform a purposeless task; for example, weeding a section of the campus where no one goes. What we are saying by requiring this is, *"Jim, you've demonstrated that you're not willing to follow the program at all, so we're going to remove you from it completely. You are in complete control over how long this will last but you have become a major burden to work with. Therefore, we're going to arrange matters in such a way that you will be a burden only to yourself."* At this point, we are looking for any sign from Jim that he sees the connection between his attitude and the meaningless nature of his tasks. This step is not one that is taken lightly. It is a clear message to Jim that he will not be permitted to make a mockery of the school and its disciplinary standards.

Taking this scenario to a final level, let's assume that while Jim was on his fourth day of **2-4** he managed to have a cigarette from a pack that he had hidden somewhere during his first few days at school. Let's also assume that he was seen smoking by the maintenance staff. This act would demonstrate that Jim saw the entire process as little more than a joke. This would demonstrate beyond a shadow of a doubt that Jim was not willing to comply with the program. Chances are there are other students in school in Jim's boat and it is for these students that the **Wilderness Outpost** has been designed.

With the Wilderness Outpost, faculty supervisors take a group of eight to twelve students to a wilderness site or perhaps an island off the coast of Maine. The students are fully equipped with supplies and camping equipment. The message that they are given is:

> *You've demonstrated that you're not going to follow the Hyde program; therefore, we'll give you a program you can follow. If you want to have a bad attitude out here, that's fine. Now only you and others in the group will suffer the consequences of your attitude. On the other hand, if you demonstrate a positive attitude and come together as a group, we will return to school soon and you will be back in the regular school program. If you continue to exhibit the attitude which brought you here, you will remain out here indefinitely. The choice is yours.*

In this instance, the faculty member's role is to provide a safe environment and to supervise a project undertaken by the group. Past groups have built campsites in the wilderness for other campers to enjoy. One summer a hiking trail that others could use for exploration was built by a group camping out on Seguin Island. The Wilderness Outpost generally lasts for a week to ten days but has been known to extend longer. It entirely depends upon the attitudes within the group.

CONCLUSION

What is the purpose of this approach to discipline? The point is simple. We believe that individuals should be accountable for their actions. A student who chooses to smoke, drink, lie or cheat has made a decision to violate the ethics he or she earlier agreed to follow. There are consequences for this decision. While this explains Hyde's standpoint from a negative view, the positive perspective is more important. We have learned that a student can't pursue his or her personal growth in earnest with a conscience anything less than clear. If a student attempts to do the Hyde program while sneaking cigarettes on the side, there is no way that he or she can ultimately succeed. Success at Hyde School requires whole-hearted commitment. We would venture that most serious endeavors in life require the same. The forward surge that a student takes after clearing his or her conscience is an inspiring phenomenon to behold. Initially, a student not only resists the opportunity to clear his or her conscience but will often protest as well. After consciences have been cleared and accountability has been served, students generally feel better about themselves. They are better equipped to pursue excellence within the Hyde curriculum.

10

Dormitories: Staffing and Rooming

by Hamilton Gregg, Director of Residence
Oregon Episcopal School
Portland, Oregon

I have spent much of my life in boarding schools, as a student, teacher and administrator. I was a country boy of divorced parents living in Aspen, Colorado. Skiing and decadence were a large part of the culture; there were too many distractions for a youngster like me who required guidelines and boundaries. So when I was ten I was shipped east from my private Country Day School to the Malcolm Gordon School, a very small, very strict boarding school of 34 students in a gorgeous Victorian mansion overlooking the Hudson River. Other than geographical proximity, there didn't seem to be much rhyme or reason to rooming assignments except that older students (eighth graders) set the example for their younger peers as roommates and were overseen by a strict dormmaster.

The switch to St. Mark's in ninth grade was a whole new world. It was friendlier, a far more connected group. A large number of students all lived in one building. Bonding was natural and welcome. Students of all ages were mixed together for rooming purposes. After freshman year we could choose room and roommates. Peer-elected senior prefects and proctors ran the dorms with dormmasters. Staff was usually young, fresh from college, wet-behind-the-ears with a keen interest in teaching, but with little training in the complexities of dealing with hormone-abundant teenagers. After four years there I was not to think about boarding dormitories for another eight years. Upon graduation from college, I tried my hand at a variety of jobs and finally decided to return to school life. I started out at The Thacher School in Southern California as associate director of admission and after three years and a master's, moved to the Oregon Episcopal School where I am now director of residence. I have been involved in residential staffing decisions and rooming assignments to varying degrees and have discovered that these should be the top priorities in a successful boarding school.

Residential Staff

Staffing is a key element in a healthy residential community. Young, enlivened college graduates come to boarding schools as teachers from all around the country hoping to affect the lives of teenagers. They are idealistic and energetic. They bring fresh thoughts to the community. Close in age to the students, they are the life blood of the prep school. They can speak the students' language. They come with high expectations and they want to be involved in every aspect of a young person's life —teaching, coaching, running activities, being dorm parents, and disseminating ethics.

Unfortunately many of the new faculty are ill-prepared for the rigors of boarding school life. They want to be friends with the kids and they do not wish to be seen as the task master or disciplinarian. They want to have freedom to play and work. Seldom are they aware of the totality of the responsibilities they are undertaking, that teaching, living and working in a boarding school is similar to entering a new culture. Each school is particular; each has its own uniqueness, history and traditions. Choosing to be a dorm parent means choosing a way of life.

Dorm parents are responsible for the lives and education of each of the students with whom they have contact. Further, many times dorm parents are *de facto* guardians. Many fail to realize that this responsibility means letting go of the freedoms with which they have become accustomed. They, too, must follow the rules of the school. For instance, if the school does not allow smoking, it is not appropriate for them to smoke on campus. For many, these constraints are difficult. Further, they are now saddled with a large group of teenagers. Most important, they often fail to acknowledge that their actions are recorded in the minds of every one of those kids. If they are not consistent in punishment, show favoritism, turn their back on infractions or major rule violations, the kids know it and respond. Boarding students not only expect dorm parents to act like their own parents but to be perfect and judicious. It is a hard role to fill.

How do young faculty get the training necessary to be effective and conscientious without abusing the privileges they feel they have so rightly earned? Dorm faculty turnover is a common occurrence in most schools. This year at OES I was one among several new faces in the dorms. It is apparent that many schools do not take the time to properly explain exactly what the job entails. I have felt this frustration throughout the year. How does one explain that a person must give up weekends to drive students to the mall to go shopping or to the movies? What about the late nights getting students to settle down after a long day? How does one explain that after the day in school is over their second job is just beginning? Certainly, telling them, coaching them and appealing to them works to a certain degree but words do not reflect the realities of dorm life.

I have found that the common denominator for success in the dorm can only be developed through time on the job. At one point this year I felt that the only people to hire were those with backgrounds in boarding school, who had either attended one or worked at one. What is more important, however, is that the incoming faculty member has that special twinkle in the eye, a deep-seated interest in working with teenagers, the inner strength and courage to constantly be in the cross-fire, a willingness to work and live with a group of individuals who will constantly look to them for guidance, structure, care and understanding. Basically, dorm parents must be selflessly committed to kids, able to forego their own interests for the good of everyone else and not burnout at the same time. It is tricky to strike a balance between giving and rejuvenating oneself. Faculty members must understand their own limitations. They need to be able to take kids on hiking trips when they would rather be alone, show compassion to flu-sick kids, read English reports when they would rather go to bed, get up to stop the water fights in the middle of a hot claustrophobic night, and spend time mending love-sick hearts. Adolescents need constant attention. Year to year things change, people change, and hence the culture of the school changes. In response, dorm parents need to be flexible and forever ready for the unexpected.

Where can people like this be found? They are out there. There are some in every boarding school and public school. Do you know them when they walk in your front door? Usually not. They are like flowers that grow in the garden. Starting as buds, they need nurturing and encouragement to become effective, concerned, caring dorm parents. They need to work the trenches to understand what it is they are undertaking. I firmly believe that dorm parents need to be involved in other aspects of school life. They need to be teachers, development and admission officers, headmasters, deans, coaches, and advisors. They need to be involved in every facet of the kids' lives. Through this role-modeling they can achieve what they came to the school for: the opportunity to change and mold young people's lives. Before my arrival at OES, only one dormmaster worked full-time at the school. Consequently, the resident advisors, as they were called, knew the students only through their limited association with the dorm. There was bonding, but the close contact, the knowledge of student affairs in school, on the sports field and in their social lives was missing. Conversely, the students did not have the chance to see the RAs teach or coach and did not have any other contact with them during the day. The advantage of the "triple threat" is the constant contact. Dorm parents can seek out their charges, greet them in the morning at breakfast, coach them in the afternoon, eat with them at dinner, and help them with their homework at night. Everyone should work, live and breathe the same air. This year OES placed school faculty and administrators in the dorms and the change has been dramatic. The students feel more comfortable and remark on the improved residential atmosphere. They appreciate having the dorm parents more accessible and more involved in their lives.

Because there are not a plethora of boarding schools on the West Coast, the genre is foreign to many parents, students and faculty. Public education is the norm and boarding schools, in general, are thought to be more for delinquent students. Because of this it is difficult to get boarding staff who understand what this culture is all about. Many schools work with anyone they can get and suffer the effects of high turnover rates. Since working in a boarding school is intense and demanding, many new faculty members do not stay long. Most faculty sign one year contracts so there is the potential for losing newly trained people at the end of that tenure.

Over the course of the year, I felt that as administrators, we did a disservice to new faculty by not providing them with the appropriate training to deal with issues regarding resident students. We hoped that their zeal would carry them through the tough times. It would make sense to spend money prior to the start of school teaching new faculty and staff the skills they will need. This would save costs incurred by having to hire a new set of teachers every year. The burn-out would be less and the faculty would be more involved and equipped to deal with the complexity of issues they confront. Without this training they can only cope; they cannot be pro-active and thrive. Most schools finance training sessions too late—after the first year and during the summer months. By then, the "wet-behind-the-ears" are beaten, bruised and worn out. Some schools, like OES, spend time during the year squeezing training in at conferences. This effort helps, but again, the cost of sending all of the faculty and staff to such events is prohibitive. Many schools can only send a few faculty. Wouldn't it be better to send all the new faculty the summer prior to their first year on the job?

Money and time are the main reasons schools do not train their new faculty members. But I think every school interested in hiring new staff should make the effort to send their faculty to training sessions on issues such as diversity, gender, counseling, drug and alcohol abuse, stress, death and dying, peer relations, First Aid, CPR and other topics that are pertinent to becoming responsible and capable dorm parents. They need this information and the students expect this type of well-prepared individual, to say nothing of what parents expect when they entrust their sons or daughters to a school.

At the beginning of each school year, prior to the arrival of the students, my staff and I spend a week preparing for the beginning-of-the-school-year rush. We discuss rules, regulations, procedures and so on. We come to a consensus on how we will apply the rules and what sort of consequences will follow when these rules are broken. Since my arrival meant an overhaul to the system, our group spent a great deal of time working out these policy decisions. But this was not enough. We were all greenhorns with our own ideas of how a dorm should run, how we should act and what our goals for the year should be. Only a few of us had had actual experience. Throughout the year, we met every Wednesday night to review the week, talk about different students, think of different ways to deal with situations, revise policies, and plan weekend activities. We found these meetings to be important for disseminating information to the whole group as well as for group support, commiseration and team building. We chatted, caught up with each other and took some time out of the week for ourselves. The meetings were so useful that I recommend that other schools make residential staff meetings part of their *weekly* schedule.

Rooming

Decisions involving roommate selection are difficult and tricky, but crucial. The Thacher School is a unique school located in a small artist/agricultural valley know as The Ojai. The school houses approximately 250 students in seven dorms spread about the campus. The dorms vary by size, sex and class. Aside from two freshman dorms, there are dorms with a mix of sophomores and juniors, and others with juniors and seniors. Thacher's rooming philosophy is different than those at other schools with which I am familiar. Freshmen are each given singles. Thacher asks a great deal of its students academically and physically, and a separate dorm allows the freshmen to bond as a group. Because most freshmen may be away from home for the first time, the school feels that they should be given the space and time to live alone and adjust to both the schedule and the school itself. When the students move along into the next grade they then have roommate and rooming choices.

As with many schools, Thacher gives seniors a great deal of responsibility in the running and management of the dorms via the position of prefect. Prefects are responsible for maintaining the decorum and atmosphere of a section of a dorm. They are expected to give out punishments, conduct room checks on weekends, organize social events, supervise evening check-in, and perform many other dorm-related activities that, at other schools, are usually reserved for the dorm parents. The punishments they can give depend on the particular dorm. One dorm gives strikes for minor offenses: dirty rooms, loud music, late for check-in and so on. Once a student receives three strikes, he or she must work for three hours around the school. This ability to give punishment adds to the respect seniors receive as long as the privilege is not abused. It also eases the prefects' job in the management of the dorm by giving them power behind the position. Finally, this role helps soften the barrier between faculty and students.

At the end of the junior year, students apply for the position of prefect in any of the dorms, each of which has a number of prefects and a head prefect. The interviewing process with each dorm head lasts for a week. A negotiation process occurs as each of the dorm heads tries to get the "best" juniors to be prefects in their respective dorms. The most responsible juniors are selected to run the freshmen dorms. The prefect's position is highly valued by the students. The selection period causes a great deal of anxiety among candidates. In fact, many sophomores choose not to become involved in School Year Abroad, Experiment in International Living or other off-campus programs for fear of being eliminated from prefect contention.

As far as perquisites go, prefects are given select rooms in the dorms. These accommodations tend to be larger and more comfortable. Some have fireplaces and each is situated in the middle of a dorm section. This way, prefects have a view of each room or at least can control the traffic through the halls.

I like Thacher's rooming policy. It allows each class to stay and live together for essentially three years while offering expanded contact with other classes. This helps the class remain unified until it assumes the responsibility of running a dorm. The system has a long tradition and it works well.

I had only been marginally involved in the process of selecting roommates until earlier this year when I became director of residence for the Oregon Episcopal School, a college preparatory school in Portland, Oregon. I have come to realize that rooming is a difficult process. It requires forethought and imagination. One has to consider the personality of each student, their neighbors and the dorm as a whole. The make-up of the dorms will have ramifications for community life.

In August my staff and I began choosing roommates for a group of students about whom we had little knowledge. We knew how crucial it is to know the students and their habits in order to assign them appropriate rooming groups. Two of the nine staff members were returning and knew the students who were also returning. We entered the process with a little mysticism and a whole lot of hope.

The process at OES is similar to that at other schools. At the end of the previous year students are asked to fill out a form that lists both rooming and roommate choices. We have had a lot of leeway in our selection process this year because, while we have room for about 70 boarders, only 45 students were to live in the dorms. But we are also constrained by the same issues that confront other schools, namely, how are we going to create a harmonious atmosphere given the composition of the student body and the configuration of rooms? In addition to meeting the rooming desires of the students, we, like our larger counterparts, must also consider details such as: boy/girl populations, dorm capacities, single vs. double rooms, and cultural issues.

The challenges that confront us are several. First, the make-up of the dorms is close to 50 percent international. We have both foreign and American students that fit that bill. Over a third of the boarding population is made up of foreign nationals from Japan, Korea, Indonesia, Thailand, Germany, India and Spain. The rest are international Americans, mostly from ARAMCO, the Arab-American Oil Company in Saudi Arabia.

This multicultural make-up provides a wonderful opportunity for students to live closely with their foreign counterparts. The students may have little idea of the value of this opportunity for them and their futures, but we, as dorm parents, must consider the implications of these demographics. We must be aware that Japanese students may not wish to live with Korean students because of their countries' age-old rivalry. We must be sensitive to language barriers. We must try to separate students from the same country especially if they have little knowledge of English. We do this in order to expand the experience of the students and force them to become less dependent on their mother tongue. We also must try to spread the leaders among the emotionally needy students in the dorm. A great deal of thought needs to be put into the process.

Over the year, it has become apparent that one must know more than personalities when putting a dorm together. For instance, this year I learned that many Asian students tend to work late at night, shower before going to bed and wake up late. This is part of their culture. The more information one has, the better one can organize the dorms.

Second, the OES dorms are comprised of two adjacent, two-story buildings, one for girls and one for boys. Each dorm has a common room, the boys with two. Each building has three faculty apartments, one at each end and one in the middle. We currently house 35 boys and ten girls. This male/female ratio is one of the major issues now confronting us. The boys dorm is larger and will always have more students and we need to keep in mind that the girls will always feel at a disadvantage, will always struggle for their voice in residential life.

Third, we do not have enough freshmen to warrant giving them their own building, floor, or section. Thus the freshmen do not have the opportunity to bond as a group and become familiar with group living before sharing a dorm with older students. The sophomores, juniors and seniors often become frustrated with them. But this rooming structure gives the freshmen the chance to integrate with the other classes and the whole dorm can bond together. No one group gets singled out. Tolerance, patience and acceptance all play a heightened part in everyone's lives on a daily basis.

Finally, one issue that I have struggled with over the year is trying to get seniors to take an active role in the running of the dorm. I value the system Thacher has implemented. Senior prefects there take their position seriously and the dorms manage themselves because of their efforts. More important, everyone is expected to be responsible and is held accountable. This year at OES I have been trying to build that kind of program. Senior responsibility plays a role in rooming because without seniors taking part in monitoring the dorm, dorm parents need to take up the slack. This is certainly part of the dorm parent's job, but without any group or person bridging the gap between the faculty and the student, a "we/they" attitude is created. Rather than being leaders in the dorm, the seniors become part of the crowd. Therefore, dorm parents need to look to those seniors who are leaders and utilize them in the rooming plan by spreading them out through the halls where they can be effective.

Throughout this winter and spring, I spent an hour every Tuesday evening discussing leadership with the seniors. We discussed why they were considered leaders, and how they, as the oldest students, could be more effective in the dorms. Most important, we talked about how seniors are viewed by the other students. If they choose not to take responsibility they are then condoning questionable behavior among the other students. Making a choice to act or not to act is a choice. Both have consequences. At times, trying to get seniors to take action feels like teaching fish to walk. This is partly due to the fact that there are no student role models for them to look to. When I talk to them about being leaders I cannot refer to any of their contemporaries. In a sense, I am working in a vacuum. I envision this process taking several years to catch on. By the time the current freshmen are seniors I hope they will know the meaning of leadership and be able to apply this knowledge in the dorm.

Having thought about the rooming process a little more than when I stepped onto the OES campus eight months ago, I can now look at it with more insight. It is worth taking the time to scope out potential conflicts before the school year begins. So this year we decided to begin the rooming process in the spring while the personalities of the kids are still fresh in our minds. Toward the end of the semester we will hand out rooming selections and make the choices before students leave for the summer. This will give those of us making up the room plan an advantage. We will remember the personalities of the students with ease. Come the end of the summer we need only place new students in the empty rooms or with returning students who chose to room with matriculating students. Finally, if problems arise they can be handled in the spring rather than in the middle of the school year.

Since we have not used this system before there will undoubtedly be unforeseen issues that arise. However, it does seem to make some sense. The idea came to me while I was at the NAIS Conference in San Francisco. I had been attending several seminars on boarding school programs, counseling, and so on. I thought about how I felt coming into a new job at the beginning of the year and how out of touch I felt with the students who were to be my charges. I also remembered how confusing it was making rooming choices in the absence of key information. In the midst of all this, it dawned on me that perhaps, if the rooming selection was done before the end of school, the process might be much easier.

One of my philosophies is not to allow students to change rooms unless it is imperative. I have found that winter seems to be the time when tolerance wanes and everyone is looking for a change. Roommates get tired of living together; tempers, in general, are short. This is exactly what occurred this year in the boys dorm. Two roommates just could not deal with one another. But in order to move one student, other students needed to be moved as well, disrupting one quarter of the dorm. Because of these disruptions, I feel room changes should be a last resort. Living and learning together is what boarding schools are all about. By not allowing room changes we teach students to confront and deal with conflict, a skill teenagers must learn.

Future years should be easier. There may be new faculty members to train, but most should know the ropes and the expectations. There will always be adjusting and flexing. Boarding programs should not be static. They need to react to each new group of students that enters the school's halls. Better yet, boarding programs should be pro-active, preparing for every circumstance. Each class that enters our school brings with it a new perspective. It is our job to create a structure that fits. This can be achieved by designing the rooming correctly and recruiting the best possible faculty. Our ultimate goal is to create a constructive environment for both students and dorm parents, one that is harmonious and conducive to study, co-existence and building the next generation of leaders.

We should not forget this last point. Students that attend boarding school, or any school, have the potential of becoming leaders. The current high school generation will have more responsibility than any before. We cannot afford to rest on our laurels. As private school tuitions continue to rise, parents will demand more for their money; they will expect the best educational experience possible. They will not accept second rate facilities, teachers, staff or decisions. It is our job not only to meet their demands but to exceed them. Hence, we need to continue to strive to make our programs better and stronger. We need to train our staff to be the best, to look for better ways to teach our students not only about English, math, history, science and language, but also about life and all of its intricacies. This is our duty.

What were once sheltered bastions of upper class society must now develop a global awareness encompassing every aspect of the "real world." This goes beyond ethnic, economic and cultural diversity. Schools must scrutinize admission and hiring policies to adapt to the changing face of society as a whole. This includes a smaller demographic base, less financial ability to pay for private education, the handicapped and other members of the public sector. Schools will need to have a willingness to accommodate and represent each of these. Further, we need to be aware of government's increasing role in how businesses and schools operate. The American Disabilities Act is a prime example. The boarding experience is forever changing. It should be our goal, as boarding schools, to meet these changes and others that come our way with conviction and seriousness of purpose.

11

Sleeping and Eating: Skills We Need to Teach

by Mark G. Timmerman, M.D.

Adolescent Wellness

I became interested in health care for teenagers while working as a teacher, coach, and dorm parent at a boarding school in New England. While serving as assistant dean of students, I was a member of the "Health Team," which consisted of those of us involved in the academic, social, psychological, and physical well-being of the community. I was struck by how interrelated these areas were, evidenced by the observation that students faltering in one of these were usually having problems in the others as well. In fact, there is evidence correlating poor health habits (i.e. sleep, nutrition and exercise) with poor performance academically and socially.

It is perhaps an interest in social and academic performance, as well as personal attractiveness, that makes teenagers very concerned about health care issues. Several recent surveys revealed that teachers and health care providers drastically underestimate the levels of interest and responsibility that adolescents possess regarding their own health. In practice, however, teenagers represent the most medically under-served portion of our population. Despite the fact that the social and physical changes of adolescence have become progressively more demanding, this is the only age group in the U.S. that has not experienced a significant improvement in health status during the past 30 years. This combination of interest and need provided hope for the success of programs designed to implement change in this area.

In order to effectively change adolescent behavior, a delicate balance must be struck between adult guidance and student participation. Teens learn best if they are allowed to make decisions regarding their education. Teens also learn well from each other, and peer counseling and instruction groups have been used with great success for many issues regrading physical and mental health.

Perhaps of greater importance, however, is the fact that youths respond more positively to measures which reduce problem behavior for both adults and children. For instance, community efforts to reduce drunken driving have been most effective when targeted at both teenagers and adults. In other words, we must consider attempts to change the culture of our schools, rather than the "subculture" created within the student bodies and dormitories of those schools.

Attempts to change specific behaviors, in fact, often simply result in a shift to a different unhealthy activity. I recall the time that those of us working in the dean of students' office "declared war" on alcohol use in the dormitories. We offered a grace period during which students could turn in their stashes of alcohol with impunity prior to a random search of rooms. We also promised stiffer punishment, i.e. fewer "second chances" for students getting caught with alcohol. The result was, indeed, a reduction in alcohol use. This was evidenced both by faculty perception and self-report student surveys. Unfortunately, the same perceptions and surveys indicated that the use of more easily hidden and undetectable drugs, such as marijuana, increased in a commensurate fashion! We apparently succeeded only in shifting the drug of choice.

Thus, it is of utmost importance that we effect change by understanding the stresses of adolescence and the ways in which teenagers attempt to deal with them. We can then help educate them about these behaviors, work to provide healthy mechanisms for coping with those stresses, and enlist their participation in the process. One of our most important missions as educators is to teach students problem-solving and decision-making skills regarding their personal hygiene, social lives, and emotional well-being, for these skills will be crucial for the remainder of their lives.

The boarding environment offers a unique opportunity to help students with these issues. The commitment that boarding faculties share toward educating the "whole" student, as well as the high frequency of contact and strong rolemodeling that exist, serve as powerful tools in shaping youngsters. Naturally, boarding school life also allows for increased contact and learning between peers. It is important for us to keep these influences in mind as we discover problematic behaviors and ways to prevent them.

Dormitory Influences

Any of us who has run a dormitory is aware of the group dynamic or "personality" that a dorm acquires over the course of a year or even throughout the years. This is, of course, partly due to the leadership styles of those supervising the dorm. For the most part, however, the peer group is the primary influence in determining adolescent behavior. While this is true for any student, it is undoubtedly a more important issue for boarding students whose family influences are diminished and whose exposure to peers increased.

Studies of college and university students suggest that social influences are very powerful within dormitories. The large group size, desire to be popular within the group, and the closeness between peers generate a strong consensus among members of a residence hall. Theories of social impact indicate that the more we value a social group, the more we are willing to be influenced by it. This is true especially in adolescence, where one of the developmental tasks is the establishment of personal identity.

Social groups such as dormitories and athletic teams therefore develop forceful social norms and the pressure toward uniformity is great. One must assume that these influences are even more intense in independent secondary schools, where competition and success is generally highly valued and rewarded.

In fact, when students experience stress or distress, they are especially open to social influences. Thus, methods of coping, both healthy and unhealthy, are easily learned and shared by members of a boarding community. Interestingly, if a behavior has some prior restraint, such as self-induced vomiting, and at the same time fulfills some need, like weight control and stress release, the likelihood of this conflicting behavior increases. These theories have been corroborated by studies such as that done in Yale dormitories in 1988, which showed that binge eating (consuming a large amount of food in a short amount of time) seemed to be an acquired pattern, learned through social controls much like any other behavior.

Coping Mechanisms

It is not clear why some students develop behaviors such as binge eating or alcohol abuse while others do not. Present theory suggests that one's character structure and self-image determine how successfully one navigates the tumult of adolescence. Regardless, it seems clear that many of the unhealthy patterns that teenagers exhibit are a response to their rapidly changing environment, and, as mentioned above, that these behaviors can be learned from peers.

As students leave home to attend boarding school, they are faced with innumerable changes and new stresses. For most, this represents a first move away from their families. Young teenagers are thrust into an environment where they must suddenly become much more self-sufficient, including making new decisions about when to sleep, how to choose the right foods, how to do laundry, and how to get along with an entirely new peer group. They often find themselves in an academic and athletic (and sometimes social) environment that is more competitive and challenging than previously. When one considers that these demands are in addition to those that are requisite for any adolescent, it is easy to understand how few students are prepared to make a smooth adjustment to a new boarding environment.

The result is a predisposition to developing unhealthy techniques for coping with these stresses. The misuse of sleep, food, caffeine, alcohol and other drugs, and sexuality are examples of behaviors to which some teens turn in an attempt to adapt to their environment. These abuses carry both positive and negative consequences, and the relative invulnerability of adolescents allows them to focus on the former and discount the latter. The peer acceptance, expression of opposition to authority, and affirmation of personal identity that might result from these behaviors takes precedence to the fatigue, malnutrition, addictions, and psychological disruption that often accompany them.

A great deal of attention has been given to behaviors such as the use of alcohol and other drugs, but these represent activities that are illicit (albeit common), and abstinence is stressed. Sleeping and eating, however, provide potential for abuses that are far more widespread, for we are all obviously involved in these behaviors on a daily basis. As basic as these activities are, they require knowledge, recognition of internal cues, and moderation (which is generally more difficult for us human beings than abstinence!). There are few adults, and fewer teenagers, who understand these functions well enough to perform them appropriately, and hence it comes as no surprise that their abuse is commonplace and perhaps "spread" amongst members of boarding school peer groups.

Sleeping

David W. was a sophomore in my Algebra II class. I was a young teacher, and perhaps overly sensitive about students dozing during classes which I tried to make as entertaining as the subject matter would allow. It therefore frustrated me that David would fall asleep almost exactly ten minutes into each of my classes. Attempts at jarring, cajoling, and even teasing him into consciousness were met with several nods and an inevitable drift back into slumber. I considered him dull and obviously lazy. Needless to say, I was intensely curious when both of his parents entered the classroom during one of our "Parents' Days." I wanted to see if he would fall asleep in their presence, and especially how they would respond. After the first ten minutes, I glanced up and to my amazement found the entire W. family fast asleep! This was my introduction to the genetic component of our Circadian rhythms, the cycles that dictate for most of us a period of decreased alertness during the middle part of each day.

Of course, students falling asleep in class (and faculty nodding off during faculty meetings!) is not uncommon. In fact, it has become the norm in our society to expect several people in any group to fall asleep when the level of stimulation is decreased. As Dr. Dement, the chairman of the National Commission on Sleep Disorders, explains in his new book, *Sleepwatchers*, this should *not* be considered normal behavior. It is rather a manifestation of the ubiquitous lack of sleep, or "sleep debt" that we have all come to accept. Stanford research subjects that received an adequate amount of sleep at night did not fall asleep during periods of decreased stimulation during the day, including the times when their individual daily rhythm alertness levels were low.

A clear relationship has been established between sleep debt and performance on tasks involving attention, memory, motor and cognitive skills. Recent accidents such as the Exxon Valdez oil spill and the explosion of the space shuttle Challenger have been linked to faulty action by individuals who were seriously sleep- deprived. In addition, sleep debt has been found to significantly potentiate the effects of alcohol, making the abuses of sleep and alcohol a deadly combination.

Due to the external demands placed on them, as well as an internal need for an increased amount of sleep, adolescents are at especially high risk for accumulating sleep debt. Dr. Carskadon at Brown University has done a number of important studies on secondary school student populations. One of the most striking findings is that students entering high school require one to two hours *more* sleep than they did as preadolescents in order to maintain the same level of daytime functioning. In spite of this, teenagers are often asked to start classes earlier, and at the same time are allowed more freedom in choosing bedtime. The result is that adolescents sleep less than preteens, go to bed at a later hour, and experience an increased level of daytime sleepiness. They receive an average of approximately seven hours of sleep, whereas they need about nine hours for optimal functioning.

The consequences of this adolescent sleep debt, which is cumulative, are manifold. Sleep deprivation has been shown to make students prone to: accidents, sleepiness in class, mood and behavior problems, decreased motivation, adverse effects of drugs and alcohol, and the development of major sleep disorders such as insomnia and narcolepsy. It seems evident, also, that immune systems are compromised by insufficient sleep, making students more susceptible to illness. In spite of this, they remain a population that is especially naive about sleep, including how much to get, how to recognize a significant sleep debt, and what the consequences of sleep deprivation are.

Perhaps this naivete is what encourages them to so readily adopt decreased sleeping time as a way to deal with the demands placed on them. Indeed, there is almost a mystique about staying up late, and my experience as a dormitory parent leads me to believe that this is especially true in the boarding school environment. Teens enjoy pushing limits, and we are all familiar with the proud yet self-pitying announcement of ''all-nighters'' that were ''pulled'' during the previous night. These behaviors are observed by others in the dorm and become the social ''norms'' of the peer group. In competitive schools, some students inevitably interpret this to mean they will not be able to make the grade unless they, too, work late into the night.

Subsequently, the use and abuse of stimulants is widespread amongst adolescents, and may be one of the habits that is most easily learned amongst members of dormitory peer groups. Caffeine is the most popular of these stimulants and is found in compounds such as Nodoz and Vivarin, as well as coffee and tea. Despite the fact that this is a ''legal'' drug, its side effects, including nervousness, irritability, and sleeplessness are more common than many of us would like to admit.

In addition, it seems that students are generally inefficient about their use of early evening hours, when socializing and procrastinatory behaviors dominate. When students really want to accomplish something, whether academic or illicit, it becomes ritual to engage in the activity late at night. During those times, the dorm is quiet and one can work privately. Most importantly for those involved in non-academic pursuits, the dormitory parents are asleep. I found, in fact, that the students in my dorm knew my routine almost down to the time I usually brushed my teeth. If I was intent on making a "bust," I would set my alarm for 2 a.m. then stroll through the corridor. It was more than once that I was greeted with the ironic question, "Why Mr. T! What are you doing up at this hour?"

Then, of course, we all are also familiar with the "ghost town" silence of weekend mornings on boarding school campuses. This "crashing" phenomenon, which has become the norm for adolescents, is simply the result of the sleep debt that students accumulate throughout the week. Unfortunately, teens shift their internal clocks as they stay up and rise late on weekends, making it difficult to fall asleep early on Sunday nights. This "Sunday night insomnia" is part of what creates the "zombie-like" expressions that teachers see as they scan their classes on Monday mornings.

Are these behaviors more problematic amongst boarding students? A study of 600 students at a New England preparatory school revealed significant differences between boarders and day students. Boarding students went to sleep an average of one hour later, on both weekdays and weekends, than their day student counterparts. Interestingly, they received approximately the same amount of total sleep because boarders were more likely to wake later, skip breakfast, and run off to class. Despite the similar total sleep time, however, a higher percentage of boarders reported too little sleep (83 percent boarders vs. 70 percent day students). I might add that these numbers indicate significant deficiencies for both groups. Boarding students were also more inclined to use caffeine daily (29 percent boarders vs. 19 percent day students), and were more prone to fall asleep in class at least once a week (18 percent boarders vs. 5 percent day students). Unless there is a qualitative difference in sleep in dormitories, Benjamin Franklin's sage adage seems to be corroborated by the above evidence.

What role, then, might curfews have in influencing sleep? In a different study of freshmen and sophomores in three New England boarding schools, 32 percent of students with curfews went to bed regularly before 11 p.m. compared to only 14 percent of students without curfews. On the average, students without curfews went to bed one hour later than those with curfews. Students with curfews behaved more like day students in the previous study, going to bed earlier and rising earlier, but getting about the same amount of total sleep. Once again, this "early-to-bed, early-to-rise" pattern was associated with far less daytime sleepiness than was found in "noncurfew" students.

Sleep, thus, seems to be an area which warrants some attention by boarding school faculty and administration. We must view sleeping as a function which requires guidance and education, especially due to our *in loco parentis* status. A successful approach might include campus-wide programs aimed at educating the community about sleep and sleep debt. Integrating the subject into the curriculum would be equally important. As much as possible, students should participate in the education process. This might even involve some groups maintaining sleep diaries, in order to learn more about their own sleeping habits and how they relate to daytime performance (i.e. grades, athletics, mood, etc.). After students understand these issues better, they may be quite willing to become involved in discussions and decisions about establishing and enforcing curfews and lights-out policies.

Because student nocturnal behavior is directly affected by dormitory supervision, this deserves important consideration, as well. When I first read the recommendations for more "full-time" dormitory faculty by Louis Crosier in *Casualties of Privilege*, I found myself defending tradition. After all, I had been a "triple threat" myself, having served as teacher, varsity coach, and full-time dormitory parent. (I also subsequently left boarding schools to go to medical school, which probably was less exhausting!). I then reminded myself about the traditional surgeon's lament: "I hate being on call every other night—that way I get to see only half the good cases." It is true that the 36 hour shifts which are common in medical internships offer excellent continuity of care, but one must question the quality of that care.

Fortunately, medical education is becoming more humane. Physicians are realizing that things don't need to be done a certain way simply because it is the way it used to be done in the "good old days." In fact, society has changed greatly in the past few decades. Our culture places more professional demands on women and more domestic demands on men. This sharing of responsibilities both inside and outside the home leads to a dynamic and fulfilling lifestyle, but it also makes it more difficult to balance the forces which compete for our time and energy. We must consider the fact that we will attract and retain well-rounded and well-adjusted individuals to demanding fields such as boarding school education and medicine only if we make allowances for sufficient family and personal time.

I, therefore, feel that some of the continuity that might be lost in taking away some of the "triple threat" responsibilities would be more than made up for by the quality of supervision that might result. When I was a dorm parent, I viewed evening hours as "no news is good news." After all, I had lesson plans of my own to prepare and I rarely ventured into the corridor unless it sounded like damage control was necessary. A full-time dorm supervisor might offer more *active* dorm parenting, including making rounds throughout study hours to assist in homework assignments and helping students use their time efficiently. This would undoubtedly make late night activity less necessary. A dorm parent without a full schedule of daytime responsibilities would also be better able to keep track of and respond to late night activities.

The evidence stated earlier suggests that such changes might allow students to learn to manage their time better, sleep more and during healthier hours, and experience improved daytime performance and well-being. We might even expect an increase in the number of students that make it to breakfast, which has been shown in several studies to improve classroom performance. This leads us to another aspect of daily lifestyle that students often abuse.

Eating

Making decisions about food is another of the many new responsibilities that students face when they leave home to attend a boarding school. In general, adolescents have extremely limited knowledge of the basic facts about nutrition, dieting, and eating disorders. In most cases, however, we open our cafeteria lines to them, somehow expecting them to figure out which types and amounts of food to consume.

Boarding schools have the opportunity, indeed the responsibility, to teach students behavior that will enable them to succeed as adults. While the high level of activity and growth of adolescents may allow their bodies to compensate for their poor dietary habits, those same nutritional patterns often carry devastating consequences later in life. If we can help students develop lifestyle patterns that will allow for the prevention of heart disease, high blood pressure, osteoporosis, obesity and other eating disorders, we will enable them to fully utilize the superlative education that private schools offer.

At the same time, the rapid growth and increased nutritional requirements of adolescents make them more susceptible to deficiencies of calories, vitamins, and minerals. Teens also readily adopt fad or vegetarian diets that may not be nutritionally sound or balanced. This is especially true for females, who are generally striving to be thin and consume fewer than the recommended calories for their weight and activity level. In addition, girls are predisposed to anemia because of menstrual blood loss and to osteoporosis due to hormonal influences. Despite this, about 50 percent of teenage girls eat less than two-thirds the Recommended Daily Allowance of iron and calcium, placing them at significant risk for these problems.

Athletes are also at increased risk for nutritional deficiencies. While they have increased energy demands, they often consume fewer calories because they tend to be body-image conscious and also as competitive about their looks as about their sport. Many sports, such as gymnastics and wrestling, also emphasize a lean body type. In addition, strenuous training leads to increased anemia and often, for girls, the loss of menstrual periods, raising the risk level for future osteoporosis and possibly even infertility for those females. Superimposing many of these factors, one can see that adolescent female athletes are at significant risk for health problems related to nutrition, and this may be even more true for students in boarding schools, who usually eat without supervision.

The dormitory is, in fact, a common place for nutritional abuse. Many of us who have run dorms have witnessed widespread consumption of snack foods, particularly late at night. Most pizza delivery persons are all too familiar with campus dormitories. Interestingly, many students who pass up dinner or eat just a salad, in an attempt to stay slim, resort to the soda, chips and candy that dormitory vending machines readily offer as hunger finally overwhelms them late in the evening. Because of the "subculture" influences of residency groups mentioned earlier, behaviors such as snacking, dieting, and even self-induced vomiting are often shared between members of a dormitory. Few students can hide these behaviors from their room- and dormmates for very long, and, while some of these activities may initially be met with disdain, girls often see the "beneficial" effects that may result, and find themselves compelled to engage.

There is evidence to support this notion that problematic eating behaviors are more common for girls living in dormitories. In a study that I performed involving four independent secondary schools with both boarding and day students, the prevalence of bulimia nervosa and other dangerous eating patterns were much higher for boarders than day students. Overall, we found approximately 15 percent of girls in grades 10-12 to be frequently engaged in drastic and dangerous eating and dieting behavior.

Thus food becomes a common abuse substance during adolescence. Approximately one half of normal weight teenage girls are actively involved in dieting at any given time. Once again, it is the stress of pubertal change, including rapid body growth, weight gain, and development of sexuality that causes students to seek coping mechanisms. Our culture rewards thinness, especially in females, and hence girls receive "positive" reinforcement for dieting, abusing laxatives and diet pills, and self-induced vomiting. This reinforcement is difficult to resist, especially for an adolescent who is, by definition, highly concerned about body shape and self-image.

Many recent studies suggest that we have become a society that is even more image-conscious than before. In fact, several authors argue that the mind-altering focus and subsequent psychotropic drug use of the 60s has shifted to one of body image and the drugs and behaviors that alter it. Of recent interest are studies that show the number of boys who abuse anabolic steroids in an attempt to become bulkier is equivalent to the number of girls who develop eating disorders in an attempt to become slimmer.

Anorexia nervosa and bulimia nervosa are the severe manifestations of eating problems that serve as maladaptive methods of coping with the crisis of adolescence. About one percent of our teenage girls develop anorexia, which is a self-starvation syndrome that produces many serious physical complications and leads to the death of ten percent of those who are afflicted. Bulimia is a binge-purge syndrome that involves about three percent of adolescent females, and is probably not quite as devastating physically as anorexia but perhaps more damaging psychologically. It is important to point out that, while three to four percent of our young women will develop these disorders (there is some overlapping of the syndromes), many more are routinely engaged in dangerous eating and dieting behaviors.

What can boarding schools do to help prevent these dangerous behaviors? As with sleep, we have an opportunity to provide information and teach behaviors that will serve our students well throughout their lives. As mentioned earlier, we might focus some attention on the stresses of adolescence, including the special stresses inherent in a boarding community, and teach students healthy methods of coping. Workshops and curricula that involve demonstration and role-playing could help develop skills in resisting peer and media influences, stress reduction, and social problem solving.

With respect to eating, we must take an active role in teaching students about nutrition and making appropriate food choices. In fact, I would suggest that one of the most important adjustments to boarding school life is learning to make healthy use of the cafeteria, and that this should be included in new student orientation.

Campus-wide attention could also be applied to education about nutrition. Programs that have been the most successful in high school environments have integrated a dynamic approach to classroom instruction, such as self-assessment, food diaries, contests, food preparation, tasting fairs, and classification of foods into "anytime," "sometimes," and "now and then" food groups. Not surprisingly, peer instruction and counseling have been important parts of effective programs.

Snacking is another area of concern, with adolescents consuming approximately 30 percent of their calories from snacks. Because this phenomenon is so pervasive, I would suggest that we simply help students snack in a healthy manner. If we encourage teens to substitute nutritionally dense foods for their empty calorie sodas and candy, we can allow snacking to be an asset rather than a liability. Healthy foods can easily be placed in vending machines around campus, and evidence suggests that students will often make appropriate choices if they have an option. In a study of six Canadian high schools, chocolate bar sales decreased 26 percent when apples were added to the vending machines, and soft drink sales dropped 42 percent when milk was added.

The dining hall can play a crucial role in this effort, as well. Virtually all our food services already offer choices that make a nutritionally sound meal possible, but need to go one step further in helping students make those appropriate choices. Meal plans with caloric and nutritional information could be posted in a visible area near the serving lines. It is especially difficult to receive sufficient amounts of some vitamins and especially iron for those eating a vegetarian diet, and meal plans and choices should be available for students who wish to eat meatless foods. I know of one girl's preparatory school that made a real commitment in this area, hiring a health food cookbook author as a consultant and subsequently offering healthy and appealing food choices, including well-planned vegetarian diets and freshly-baked whole grain breads.

As in the case in the dormitory, *active* supervision of students seems essential in the dining hall. While I realize that few faculty members relish the thought of sitting at the head of a table at the end of a day already filled with student contact, guidance of food choices and observation of eating behaviors is an extremely important responsibility. This is especially true when one considers that students with eating disorders very rarely are able to eat a normal meal, and hence are often easily identified by an astute observer. Schools should strongly consider holding as many "formal" meals as possible. This may be more acceptable to faculty if they have fewer dorm responsibilities, or, on the other hand, table coverage might be one of the duties given to a full-time dorm parent.

Similar attention must be placed on education about eating disorders. Students need to learn about normal physical changes of adolescence, such as the fact that by the age of 20, girls *normally* have twice as much fat and two-thirds as much muscle as boys. They should also understand that we all have a genetically determined body type, and that attempts to change it, especially without exercise, will be futile. We somehow have to find a way to build adolescent self-esteem and encourage teenagers to feel good about themselves at their normal weights.

School faculty and health center personnel need to become educated about eating disorders and how to recognize them. There should be well-established reporting and referral mechanisms in place when problems come to the attention of faculty. Health centers might consider screening instruments or even routinely examine students for weight, blood pressure and pulse, which would uncover those with more significant problems. School-sponsored programs to help overweight students lose weight sensibly have proven safe and effective. As with other aspects of changing adolescent behavior, school-wide seminars, lectures, and discussions, as well as student participation in preventative measures, will likely yield the best results.

Conclusion

Adolescents, especially those in boarding school environments, eat and sleep poorly. They are as unprepared to make responsible decisions regarding these behaviors as they are to design their own academic curricula. Because of this and the typical tumult of adolescence, they often develop abuses of food and sleep as misguided attempts to cope with their environment. Educators and health care professionals must look at ways to help students learn healthy lifestyles and constructive methods of dealing with stress. In the case of boarding communities, consideration should be given to changes in dormitory and dining hall supervision in order to facilitate these goals. Campus-wide educational programs, including student participation, would further serve to increase the effectiveness of this mission.

REFERENCES

Canadian Pediatric Society, "Adolescent Nutrition: Fast Foods, Food Fads and the Educational Challenge," *Canadian Medical Journal*, October 1, 1983, 129: 692-695.

Carskadon, M. "Patterns of Sleep and Sleepiness in Adolescents," *Pediatrician*, 1990, 17: 5-12.

Carskadon, M. "Sleep Habits in High School Adolescents: Boarding vs. Day Students," *Sleep Research*, 1988, 17:74.

Crandall, C. "Social Contagion of Binge Eating," *Journal of Personality and Social Psychology*, 1988, 55;4: 588-598.

Crosier, L. *Casualties of Privilege*, Avocus Publishing, Washington, D.C., 1991: 147-153.

Dement, W. *The Sleepwatchers*, Portable Stanford Book Series, Stanford, CA, 1992.

Hurrelmann, K. "Health Promotion for Adolescents: Preventative and Corrective Strategies against Problem Behavior," *Journal of Adolescence*, 1990, 13:231-250.

King, A., et al. "Promoting Dietary Change in Adolescents: A School-based Approach for Modifying and Maintaining Healthful Behavior," *American Journal of Preventative Medicine*, 1988, 4;2: 68-74.

Marino, D. and King, J. "Nutritional Concerns During Adolescence," *Pediatric Clinics of North America*, February, 1990, 27;1: 125-139.

Sobal,et al. "Health Concerns of High School Students and Teachers' Beliefs about Student Health Concerns," *Pediatrics*, February, 1988, 81;2.

Timmerman, M. and Wells, L. "Bulimia Nervosa and Associated Alcohol Abuse among Secondary School Students," *Journal of the American Academy of Child and Adolescent Psychiatry*, 1990, 29: 118-122.

Timmerman, M. "You Are What you Don't Eat: Our Culture's Contribution to the Development of Eating Disorders," *CWIS Newsletter*, NAIS Publications, Winter, 1992.

Truswell, A. and Darnton-Hill, I. "Food Habits of Adolescents," *Nutritional Reviews*, February 1981, 39:2 73-88.

12

Dormitory Prefects: Making a Difference, Defying the Odds

by Susan Graham, Head
The Gunnery
Washington, Connecticut

There is no comparison between life as a dorm director working with trained student leaders and life as a dorm director without. In 1977, a somewhat experienced teacher but a rookie in residential life, I accepted a job in a boarding school, assuming responsibility for a girls' dorm as well as for a full-time teaching load. I remember the high anxiety of September as I set out to manage the social and emotional lives of 55 ninth- through twelfth-grade girls—and a troubling series of incidents that followed that year in which crisis commanded our attention and "reaction" was necessarily the response. As adults, those of us in charge had little counseling experience. Those students in leadership roles in the dorm had been cast into the role simply by virtue of seniority. Expectations of the adults were vague; expectations of the students unrealistic. "Kill your own snakes," responded the administration whenever challenged by those of us in the trenches. It was a struggle to collaborate with others. There was no mental health professional or counseling team with whom to check perceptions. Weak communications between the academic and residential arenas of the school precluded any credible sequence to a student's life. What came down was often without warning—and certainly without thoughtful, predictable response. We were not even meeting the kids halfway. It was a random system and the risk was high.

It was not long before it became clear to me that there was an implicit need for a structured program—for a curriculum to direct the after hours energy and provide form and content beyond the classroom. That was 14 years ago. Since then, much of what I set out to accomplish as a teacher, counselor and dean has involved student leadership and its integration into a boarding school community. We know that what happens in dormitories affects what happens in class, in community government, on the playing fields, and surely will affect the men and women the boys and girls will become.

A commitment to hire and train the very best professionals comes first: people with "high bandwidth" as Bill Gates would say, individuals who are authentic and accessible. As Michel de Montaigne said, "Choose a guide with a well-made rather than a well-filled head. It is the achievement of a lofty and very strong soul to come down to a childish gait and guide it." The following criteria can often be helpful in considering candidates: 1) try to create a mix of married and single people; 2) insist on previous experience with kids as camp counselors, tutors, etc; 3) make sure they can drive a van—or are willing to learn! Ted Sizer once said to the Andover Board of Trustees, "House counseling is the most sophisticated, demanding academic job on this campus. Unless a student is "together" in the dormitory, his or her French or algebra or history or field hockey will suffer. . . . House counseling isn't merely supervision—it's education . . . it is a central part of the fabric of this institution . . . . Accessibility, caring, sensitivity, genuine interest, the courage to be condemnatory, to be the taskmaster or mistress as well as the readiness to be a friend: these qualities can't be categorized by "hours on duty" or items on a list to be checked off. But they are the heart of a good residential education."

Although I do not believe that dormitory personnel must have academic credentials in counseling, I do believe that they should have a "counseling orientation." Carefully structured interviews with administrators, counselors and current dormitory staff should highlight key factors essential to success in working with students in dorms. Interview questions concerning a candidate's childhood and family often reveal important attitudes about children, schooling, family values, etc. As I mentioned before, previous experience in a residential program for students—as a camp counselor or a residence hall leader in college—can save hours of orientation regarding the "spirit" of the job as well as the quality of life which it presupposes. If, in fact, a candidate has neither experience nor education in counseling or adolescent development, I encourage either summer work in a graduate counseling program or attendance at the Milton Workshop for new teachers and some focused reading from a bibliography. I highly recommend that every new member of the residential team attend the Northfield Mount Hermon Counseling Institute or the House Valley Counseling Institute, after a year "in the trenches."

A Dormitory Staff Handbook is a must, either under separate cover or as part of the Faculty Handbook. The responsibility of the dean, it should be considered a working document, reviewed and updated annually.

Dormitory directors should have scheduled meetings with the dean at least twice a month. The full dormitory staff should meet monthly. These meetings should not be seen as "extra" and squeezed into late nights, but should be legitimate staff meetings, honored by the administration. Open forums are invaluable, although structured presentations by outside professionals on relevant topics such as stress, substance abuse, eating and/or sleeping disorders, and psychological distress signals should occur once a term. What is the latest thinking on adolescent development? And what are the latest trends? Working closely with college deans often provides valuable insight into how to improve our programs. Having a "guest dean" describe the college dormitory scene can offer opportunity for discussion on how we are preparing our students to assimilate into college successfully. Continuing professional development should remain an administration's highest priority to acknowledge residential programs and to ensure the highest performance possible among the personnel designing and implementing them.

A process to select appropriate student leaders needs to begin in early spring. Sophomores and juniors should be offered the opportunity to apply in writing. A questionnaire developed by the dean of students with input from the dormitory directors offers applicants a chance to be drawn out on issues of experience, extra-curricular commitment anticipated in the coming year, changes recommended in the program, etc. This application form should be read and signed by the current dormitory staff, the student's advisor, the dean of students and the academic dean. Sessions then can be scheduled for personal interviews with every applicant. These are easiest done in clusters with interviews of 10-15 minutes back to back. A simple rating scale can help to document reactions to the students. A committee of three or four current dorm directors and three or four current prefects provides the best forum in which to conduct these interviews and eventually make the final recommendations.

Once the prefects have been selected, a week-end workshop—8-10 hours— dedicated to leadership training should ensue. In our school, it begins on Saturday evening with a wonderful meal in a special place. We use the "power room" on campus, an attractive and comfortable space reserved for only the faculty, the board of trustees and the community council. Carefully crafted to build group unity, establish open lines of communication and engender trust, a series of exercises and discussions led by the adults responsible for the group (the dean and a counselor) should be designed. The first session is time alone for the outgoing prefects to meet with the incoming prefects. Next should follow a simple ice breaker (see "Prefect Bibliography" at the end of the chapter), followed by an introduction to the workshop clearly outlining the goals. Using a film such as "The Great Santini" or "Dead Poets' Society" to examine leadership styles and coping strategies, offers an effective way to grab attention and ensure a good initial discussion. An interesting follow-up often involves the students in a self-rating inventory, revealing their own concepts of themselves and their leadership styles.

Sunday morning we begin early. Continental breakfast is followed by a session on expectations for the year ahead. I often ask them to write three goals and three fears on a piece of paper and seal it in an envelope with their name on it. Reviewing these in the middle of the next year will offer insight and valuable reflection. The dean should speak about confidentiality and establish the ground rules for the year ahead. Three other exercises usually complete the workshop. There are a myriad to choose from. My advice is that each one should be effective for the leaders—a known quantity—to set a tone and to establish a theme with the group. The theme can be reintroduced over the summer in a letter and tied into opening exercises in the fall as the group comes together to begin their work in earnest.

Our prefect system involves weekly meetings. Since prefects must negotiate the bottom-line discipline in the dorms and work with an "after hours curriculum," meeting regularly and responsibly is imperative. Ours is a dinner meeting every Monday night. It includes a variety of formats—the weekend is reviewed and the week ahead previewed, disciplinary actions are discussed, topics of concern are raised, or brainstorming sessions are led by the dean. Often guest speakers address issues which the group as a whole is struggling with: time management, crisis counseling, decision making, personal safety, recycling, consensus building, troublesome personalities or friendships, and the stresses of dual roles. There are times when the prefects themselves need attention. The time prior to holidays or exams is a pressure cooker for them as they try to manage their peers' lives and their own. Often devoting an hour to their issues, usually generated by exhaustion and the ambivalence of being caught between adult authority and student suspicion of it, can be invaluable. Open discourse with trusting adults who are good listeners is imperative if dorm prefects are to be successful. These are the kids on the front lines and they must be able to check their perceptions with professionals who are sensitive to their needs and clear about signals.

Additional time to gather the prefects alone with the staff is an invaluable booster to both morale and performance. It should be scheduled at least twice during the school year. Sometime in the fall, plan to get them all off campus for a day on an adventure course. Local campuses offer the best opportunities. Physical experiences designed to enhance group dynamics, trust, and coopera-tion add a heightened sense of ownership to the group and increase the confi-dence quota of everyone. I recommend October; the students will have had some time "in the trenches" and the weather should still be wonderful. The end of January can be a very vulnerable time. Spirits are low, seniors are beginning to become disenfranchised and the midwinter slump is settling in. Again, get them off campus for an overnight to reflect on where they have been as well as where they are going and to let them have some fun together. Feedback, celebration and friendship should be the focus.

Acknowledging and training the students who are willing to risk the possibil-ities and attendant responsibilities of leadership is one of the most important aspects of any residential program. These are volatile, intense, complicated years, rife with dimensions involving friendship/achievement, work/love, competence/conscience. We hold high expectations of our students. That they attend to their academics goes without question. But there is so much more beyond the classroom. I believe that it's important for as many students as possible to experience leadership, to consider critically the complex human dilemmas presented by the world which they will soon inherit, to go beyond narrow convergent thinking and see relationships and connections in their community as being of paramount importance to the service of a better world.

SAMPLE LEADERSHIP MATERIAL

Prefect Job Description

You will be responsible:

1. For meeting with the students in your dorm regularly—both in group meetings and one on one.
2. For possibly another class period for learning counseling skills.
3. For attending a processing meeting once a week with your dorm director.
4. For attending approximately two evening workshops:
   Spring Leadership Training
   The October and January Leadership Conference
5. For remembering that you are a ''role model.''
6. For accepting your year long commitment through good times and through all other times.

Source: S. R. Powell

Prefect Application

1. Participation in the leadership training program requires enthusiasm, responsibility, dedication, and a desire to help others. Describe what you think you can contribute to this program.
2. Why would you want to be a prefect? Explain what you think you would gain.
3. What do you think the other students might gain from your leadership?
4. If your best friend were asked to describe what type of person you are, what five words would he/she use.
   1.   4.
   2.   5.
   3.
5. List your hobbies and extracurricular activities.
6. What academic commitments will you have next year?
7. Complete the following sentence: I would most like to be remembered for:

Source: S. Graham/S. Langan

Evaluation of the Prefect Leader Applications

1. On the written application each question will be worth ten (10) points. One (1) would be a score given if the response was deemed to be inappropriate or unacceptable. Ten (10) would be a score given if the response was absolutely outstanding and without fault. Use a sliding scale between 1 and 10 to evaluate each question.
2. You will be asked to rank each applicant during the group meeting on the following qualities. Since it would be unfair to write or take notes during the group process meeting, have these qualities in mind and be an excellent observer. Again the ranking will be on the sliding scale 1-10.
   1. Enthusiasm
   2. Sincerity, openness, willingness to give and connect
   3. Ability to interact with group members
   4. Ability to listen

Source: S. Graham/S. Langan

Biographical Interview

GUIDELINES FOR INTERVIEWING

1. Face your partner.
2. Show genuine interest, both verbally and non-verbally.
3. Don't interject your own opinions or experiences while interviewing.
4. Take brief notes.
5. Paraphrase occasionally to make sure your understanding is accurate.
6. Give your partner plenty of time to respond to each question.
7. Make it clear at the start that your partner may pass on any question (not answer), or come back to it later if preferred.

QUESTIONS

1. What are 3 things you like to do? Why?
   a. _____
   b. _____
   c. _____
2. Where did you grow up?
   _____

   What was the best thing about growing up there? _____

3. Think for a moment about the persons who have influenced the kind of person you are today—parents, teachers, family, friends. What person or persons stand out as having the greatest influence? Why? _____

4. What is something you have done, accomplished, or become of which you are proud? _____

_____

5. What is a way you would like to grow, personally or professionally, during the coming year? _____

_____

6. What are some of your expectations for the workshop? _____

_____

Source: T. Likona

Student Leaders' Workshop

EXPECTATIONS

1. What do you expect from yourselves as proctors/prefects?
2. What do the students expect from you?
3. What does the school expect from you?

CONFIDENTIALITY

1. Who has it?
2. Who doesn't?
3. When can you keep a secret?
4. How can you avoid saying you will when you can't?
5. What can you say to help a student?

SURVIVAL

1. What do you need to survive this year?
2. What do you need to survive this week?
3. Who will you ask for help?
4. How will you ask for help?
5. Why are proctors often afraid to ask for help?
6. Who/What are your support systems?
7. How do you create them?
8. How do you know if you are doing a good job?

Source: B. Sherwood/S. Graham

Styles of Leadership

1. Think of a person who, in your opinion, is a competent, effective, successful leader. What qualities and/or skills does this person exhibit/use (name at least three) which cause you to consider him or her a ''good'' leader?

2. Think of a person who, in your opinion, is not a competent, effective, successful leader. What are the problems with this person's behavior or attitude (or whatever) (name at least three) which cause you to consider him or her a "less than good" leader?

3. Briefly describe a situation involving at least one other person in which you were expected or chose to play a leadership role. State the context, player(s), task(s)/goal(s), and outcome(s) of the situation.

What qualities or skills did you exhibit/use which helped you to act and be perceived as a competent, effective, successful leader (name at least three)?

What were the problems (name at least three) which contributed to your inability to act and be perceived as a competent, effective, successful leader?

What things do you still need to work on?

Source: S. Moore

Letter to Coordinator of the Prefect Program

Dear:

Your continuing role as coordinator of the prefect program builds consistency and quality into what I consider to be one of our most crucial programs. The rewards for all involved are multidimensional and their cumulative effect in the realms of enhanced communication, self confidence, and relationships among peers surely make a difference. Thank you for all of your efforts. Know that I appreciate them and am anxious to continue building upon our success to date.

I'd like to establish a curriculum to structure the program and to provide some bench marks for evaluation and future development. Having guidelines will help us alternate task and processing as we progress through a sequence of skill building and group bonding. My shelves are filled with resources to compliment yours and my files have been updated for 1992-93. Two or three structured activities per month, directly supervised by you is my goal for this next year. I've found that having the prefects keep journals not only facilitates quick review of the strengths and weaknesses of each exercise but also serves as a springboard for planning.

Following is a breakdown of what I see as the critical issues which we need to cover.

I. Create project hall display
   (complete by 9/15)
   Banners, murals, collages "announcing themselves"

II. Ice Breakers
New Games
Verbal, non-verbal exercises

III. Communications
Listening, paraphrasing
Emotional risk statements
Rumors exercise
Consensus building, "saying no"

IV. Self-Esteem
Self-assessment inventory
Proud whip exercise

V. Managing Stress
Self-rating
Learning to relax
Stress shield/juggler exercise

VI. Relationships
Birth order certificates
Friendship
Human bonding
Straw towers

VII. Decision Making
Styles of decision making
Auction game
Survival on the moon
Dilemma discussions
Values rating
Group dynamics
Negotiating

Needless to say, attempting to cover it all is ambitious and certainly we have to be sensitive to the rhythm of the kids' needs. From time to time, conflict resolution or crisis mediation will command the focus of the weekly meetings. But when possible, I'd like to stay on schedule and build in an appropriate evaluation so that we can continue to move ahead with insight and positive energy.

Source: S. Graham

Prefect Bibliography

D'Andrea and Salovey. *Peer Counseling Skills and Perspectives.* Science and Behavior Books, Palo Alto, CA, 1983.

Egan, Gerald. *Exercises in Helping Skills.* Brooks Cole Publishing Co., Monterey, CA, 1985.

Fluegelman, Andrew. *The New Games Book.* Headlends Press/Doubleday, Garden City, NY, 1976.

Myrick, Robert D., and Tom Erney. *Youth Helping Youth: A Handbook for Training Peer Facilitators.* Educational Media Corp., Minneapolis, MN, 1985.

Poe, Susannah Grimm, Charles Green and Tom Terrenzi ed. *Horizons.* Summit Center for Human Development, Clarksburg, W.Va., 1987.

Powell, Sharon Rose Ed.D. *Peer Group Handbook: Peer Leadership Training Exercises.* Princeton Center for Leadership Training, Princeton, NJ, 1988.

Tindell, Judith A. Ph.D. *Peer Power: Becoming an Effective Peer Helper.* Rohen and Associates Publications, St. Charles, MO, 1985.

13

To New Dorm Faculty

by Louis M. Crosier

Working in the dormitory can be the greatest experience of your life. I loved it, but I was a bit worn out after my first year. There are high points like you have never experienced and there can be low points which sneak up on you when you're not expecting them. If you plan ahead, however, these lows can be minimized.

At many boarding schools the hiring and interview process can be pretty informal. You may want to ask and answer several more questions before you start. Some of these may become real issues for you and the kids might put you on the spot with their own questions, so you should practice. Start by answering some of the following:

- What will you tell students about yourself? What will you keep private?
- What do you feel are the characteristics of an effective role model?
- What does professionalism mean to you?
- Have you ever had a crush on someone younger than you? How will you keep from becoming romantically involved with a student?
- How do you plan to create an environment in your dorm where sexism, racism and humor at the expense of others are unacceptable?
- How will you ensure that all the kids in your dorm have friends?
- How do you plan to see that all your dorm students are getting enough sleep and eating properly?
- Have you ever used drugs? How do you feel about drugs now?
- What will you do if a student approaches you with a concern but will only tell you in strict confidentiality?

These were some of the tougher questions I encountered during my first year in a dorm. But the issue which really hit home centered around a strange feeling I had about a month into school: I felt as though I had I missed my twenties. Coming from college, where I really didn't have to look out for anyone but myself, I suddenly felt like a parent of teenage kids! At first I felt accountable to my students' parents and the school, but after the first month I felt a personal obligation to the kids. I had grown to care about them and they seemed to need me. That was the weird part; they really looked to me for answers to hard questions. I sometimes wanted to say, "Hey, I'm only 22." But I got used to it and grew up quickly.

Relationships with Students

Chances are, the students will look up to you because you are older and you represent power. You can do a lot of things they can't. You will be viewed as smart because you are a teacher and "cool" because you are young. These initial assumptions on the part of the students give you a unique opportunity to have a very positive effect on their lives—their study habits, interests and self-esteem. They will probably listen to you more readily than to their parents. If you take the time, you will foster a valuable relationship and you will benefit indirectly as you help them grow, succeed and learn from their mistakes. They will be curious and ask you a lot of personal questions. In the beginning they will be your friend, but they will test you to find out whose "side" you are on—theirs or the faculty's!

Resist the temptation to be "friends" with your students. They aren't ready for your side of the give and take. If they get frustrated that you don't share your personal life, explain why, and keep it all above board. Creating distance on personal issues may be frustrating to you, but it's particularly important for young faculty who are only a few years older than the students.

If you are a young male faculty member you should be very careful of the message you send the girls. The older girls in particular may develop a romantic interest in you. They are looking toward college; they mature faster than boys. They are a sophisticated lot, looking for signs that they are attractive to men. If you are not careful about establishing a strong social life for yourself outside the school or with other faculty, you might find the attention of these girls more appealing than you should. You may want to feel young and swinging; they will want to feel sophisticated. This is a formula for potential disaster. I remember several occasions when I was a student when my female friends would talk about a teacher they thought was "hot" and they would compete for his attention. Occasionally they would "succeed" and make out or, in worse cases, have sex with him. That can have a devastating, permanent impact on an adolescent's psyche and faculty member's career and disrupt a tightly knit community more than you might imagine. I don't mean to overstate the obvious, but it is an easy trap into which even the brightest have fallen. Young female faculty, gay male and female faculty should also be careful of the messages they send the students, but historically, more inappropriate relationships develop between young male faculty and older female students.

There are many ways to avoid inappropriate relationships with students. The best way to begin is with an awareness that this is a pretty common problem. Beyond that you should be careful of when and how you use physical contact. Some is appropriate, and it will be different for kids whose families, circumstances and cultures interpret touch in a variety of ways. What to an adult is a pat on the back or a touch on the arm can mean a lot of different things to a teenager. If you find yourself spending a lot of time with a particular student ask yourself: "Am I playing favorites?" and "Who is benefiting from this relationship?" Of course, there will always be some students with whom you find it easier to establish a rapport, with whom, all things being equal, you would rather spend your time. But when you are a dorm parent it is inappropriate for these preferences to surface. Especially when you are young, you must be on your guard and resist your natural tendency to seek out those people who you sense could be your friend. If honest self-evaluation reveals that you have been favoring a student, then it's pretty late in the game, and it's better to hurt feelings earlier than later. Get advice from your faculty mentor.

If you find yourself alone with a student in any context, ask yourself what you're doing. Chances are, you're fine, but it is still important to ask yourself, to continuously evaluate. I once had lunch with a dean who told me she never went off campus with only one student. "People talk, and gossip can be nearly as harmful to a student (and to you) as being involved in an inappropriate relationship." Don't overdo it, but be careful. It gets easier as you get older or if you are married, but you're not immune. If you see one of your colleagues falling into an damaging relationship, ask him or her some of the same questions—it will be hard, but you will be doing both the student and faculty member a great favor.

On the flip side you can create a healthy relationship by serving as "coach," someone who holds students accountable and teaches them to set limits and goals for themselves. It is helpful to organize group activities within and between dorms. These might include fireside chats with guest speakers (parents with a special area of expertise), basketball, frisbee or board games, knitting or other crafts. All of these and spending time in the dorm common area to help with homework provide an opportunity to get to know your students, to model supportive behavior and to get a sense of who is fitting in and who may need help making friends.

Relationships with Colleagues and Mentors

First you need to find a mentor, or several, in whom you can confide, whose judgment you trust, and to whom you can look as a model of professionalism. You may get the best results if you tell them you would like them as your mentor and would like to meet with them regularly to discuss how you are doing. If youwork at a school with a formal mentor program, the asking step is taken care of, but be sure you feel comfortable with the mentor the school chooses for you. The key is to get frequent feedback. Regular evaluations are one of the best ways to improve your effectiveness as a teacher and dorm director. You will have to really insist on regular evaluations because they are one of the first things to go when time gets tight. Evaluations can be difficult: you may feel you have let someone down, that your job may be threatened, that you disagree with the criticism or that the demands are so unreasonable that you cannot live up to the expectations. They can also be hard for the evaluator who does not want to make you feel uncomfortable, hurt your feelings or threaten your professionalism. The best way to address these anxieties on both sides is to have biweekly two-way evaluations where both parties evaluate each other. The more often you meet, the more comfortable both parties become and the less time there is for issues to build up or escape your mind. Once you get beyond the anxiousness, there is no better way to improve your effectiveness and feel valued in your work. In addition to regular evaluations, you should have at least one formal evaluation in each of your areas of responsibility annually.

You're the new kid on the block and you should be accordingly deferential, regardless of how right you feel you are. New ideas can be quite threatening in schools where status quo is often as important as tenure and autonomy. You may be regarded as naive or idealistic. That's OK. But don't give up on the ideas about which you feel strongly. If you ask for ''advice'' and make suggestions cautiously, picking your issues, you will gain the respect of your colleagues over time. There is no overnight Wall Street success in teaching because the criteria on which you are measured have a fuzzy bottom line.

Making Time For Yourself

It's easy to let yourself get caught up in the pace of the school. You will never get bored. But it's important that you make time for yourself. You should spend time on activities unrelated to the school and you should get off campus as frequently as possible. It's important that you have people outside the prep school world with whom you can talk regularly. As the semester gets more hectic, you will find it harder and harder to make time for yourself. But you must.

During my first year as a dorm faculty member, I spent a lot of my off-duty time on campus. I ate in the dining hall and worked out in the gymnasium, but I was approached so often with school-related questions that I no longer had a life of my own. I enjoyed my students so much that I wanted to spend more time with them, but after several months it became clear to me that this benefitted no one. I was using students as a social outlet and that was inappropriate. I decided to change my routine.

To find time for myself, I scheduled blocks in which I would let NOTHING get in the way of a planned activity. My girlfriend and I went out every Tuesday night. It didn't matter where, we just left campus and spent the evening together. On Wednesday mornings from 9 to 10 a.m. I wrote letters to friends and family. On Friday mornings I'd go running for two hours from 9 to 11. That was my time and I used it to think about my life and issues unrelated to school. That's really all the time I had, but because it was scheduled, I felt in control. My girlfriend and I never missed the Tuesday evening together. On my other off-duty nights I sometimes had friends come to my apartment or I had an early dinner and read in bed. I didn't answer the door; I had a clear policy with students that I could only be disturbed in case of an emergency. "Emergency" was clearly defined, too. The students respected my request because I explained it at the beginning of the school year and because I had a "Time Off" sign on the door, unlike during my first year. I now rarely had contact with students when I was off duty. I didn't eat in the dining hall or use the campus facilities, except after hours. Finally, I kept a journal. This was my internal time. I took fifteen minutes three nights a week to write down my thoughts. It was interesting to read the journal a few months later. As with my other off-duty activities, I had a rule that I didn't write about anything school-related. Ensuring that my girlfriend and I had time for ourselves enabled me to feel fresh whenever I was on duty, so I could get involved and fulfill my responsibility to the students with no resentment.

Training and Ongoing Professional Development

After my first year of working in a dorm, I attended a boarding school conference which invited new and experienced faculty to address a variety of issues on boarding school life. It was wonderful. Through role-playing and group discussions we covered issues including: strategies for working effectively with students in the dorm and for safeguarding your personal time, raising children on campus, student-faculty intimacy, and financial planning. There, before my eyes, scenarios with which I had struggled the previous year were played out and discussed in detail. I remember thinking to myself, "I wish I had gone to this conference last year." The point is, I didn't know what to expect my first year on the job. A few days at a conference would have made the year healthier for me and my students. I think off-campus training with peers from other schools should be mandatory for all new faculty.

Of course there are a lot of other ways to stay sharp. Schools differ tremendously in what they provide their faculty in terms of in-services, outside speakers, role play work and how closely they monitor the mentor program. I found my best resource was the co-director of my dorm. We talked very honestly about issues. We passed a dorm log back and forth to keep each other up to date on what happened the night when the other was on duty. We also used this log to raise questions about how to handle certain situations with students and to discuss residential policy. We worked closely as a team even though we had little face to face contact.

Know The Resources Available To You

One of the first things I should have done when I moved into a dorm was to make a list to post by my telephone. It would have extended beyond the usual emergency numbers. I would have also included all beeper numbers for the nursing and counseling staff, security and deans' phones, all other dorm faculty numbers, the library, dining hall and maintenance. It's important to know how to reach these people after hours, on weekends and holidays as well.

You must know the procedures for handling a wide range of academic and counseling situations you may encounter during the year. Whenever you find yourself in a spot which makes you feel uncomfortable you should have a procedure for handling it. I remember a time when I was aware of one of my students staying up very late night after night. This is not uncommon at boarding school, but this student seemed particularly run down. I approached her and asked what was up. She said she had a lot of work at that time and that things were fine, "just tired, that's all." I thought little else of it and didn't pursue the matter. A few weeks later she started to go to bed earlier again.

I was lucky. A seemingly innocuous situation can sometimes be more serious. Often several faculty members will have a piece of information, a "red flag," but not think to bring it to others' attention because it seems so small. Together, these pieces can paint a picture of a student who could use some help getting back on course. I should have at least mentioned the student's fatigue to her advisor who could have checked with teachers and coaches to see if they had noticed anything unusual. At my school, the academic dean served as the information clearing house for academic matters and the dean of student life, for social and emotional concerns. The deans worked with the counseling staff, the advisor and, of course, the parents. The dorm faculty members' role was to serve as part of the information chain and, when appropriate, to work with the student on the issue of concern. But the faculty member wasn't expected or supposed to coordinate the process. A faculty member should feel free to approach a student with an issue but should also bring it to the attention of the advisor or corresponding person at the school. Sometimes, if information is kept to oneself or a situation handled unilaterally by the dorm faculty member, he or she may enable a student or colleague to continue a dangerous behavior and may in fact make it worse by tacitly condoning it.

* * * * * *

Some people say running a dorm requires frequent judgment calls. They say there's a lot of gray area for you to sift through and mistakes will happen. I'm not sure I agree with this attitude which provides an excuse for mistakes. Good training and a knowledge of the full range of resources to help with your judgment calls will erase much of the gray area. Collectively the faculty within a school have the answers to most of the problems which elude individual members. The key is to reach out to colleagues.

14

Junior Boarding Schools

by Peter P. Drake, Head
The Bement School
Deerfield, Massachusetts

I have grown accustomed to receiving skeptical looks from people when they hear that my school accepts boarders at the junior high level. They generally are curious yet polite as they inquire how any parent could send a child away at such an early age. When they pursue the issue and I explain that we sometimes accept children as early as grade 3 or 4, they become downright incredulous.

Long ago I stopped being defensive about taking boarders in grades 3-9. The vision that most people conjure is that of a nine- or ten-year-old being torn away from a warm loving family situation and thrust into an "institutional" setting devoid of family comforts and the emotional foundation that accompanies a conventional home situation. Unfortunately, the word "conventional" cannot be used to describe the family unit in the United States during the 90s. It is this fact that gives our boarding situation its validity.

What circumstances justify sending children to boarding school before they reach their teenage years? The reasons range from family instability to an unsatisfactory living environment to poor local school systems. Divorce or tragic loss of a parent can often create the type of situation that leads a family to consider the junior boarding route. Or a child might not be developing proper self-esteem within the family unit due to sibling rivalries, or he may demonstrate an inability to relate to one or both parents. In another situation the parents may be professionals and the child is cared for by a hired nanny or other live-in help. Or, a child is left alone at home for a large stretch of time in the afternoon following school. Yet another scenario has a child enduring a mediocre school circumstance which lacks challenge or the opportunity to develop academic talents. Today there are also an increasing number of American families stationed overseas who yearn for an educational opportunity for their children that can be attained in the States. The most recent phenomenon is the interest of international students, and particularly those from Asia.

I am often struck by the stereotypes that people hold regarding the types of children that attend junior boarding schools. The perception is that the boarding population is comprised solely of wealthy children whose parents don't have time for or interest in them. The truth, in fact, is that my school and most junior boarding schools are comprised of children from very diverse socio-economic backgrounds. At one time a predominant number of boarding students came from wealthy families. Now, however, that is no longer the case for junior boarding schools. One of the valuable elements of boarding is learning to live with and understand children of different cultures. In a junior boarding environment, this happens much more comfortably than at the secondary level. Children who are younger are generally more accepting of cultural differences. There is no better way to learn tolerance and understanding than by working and playing side by side without the interferences and prejudice of parents, a generation removed, who lacked a comparable opportunity.

For minority students at junior boarding schools, it is an opportunity to gain trust and confidence in a less stressful social environment. I have observed that, at the secondary level, the minority students, whether black or Asian, tend to move in tight groups and seem preoccupied by seeking their own identity rather than mixing comfortably with the other students. Our own 9th graders, when visiting secondary schools for future placement, have often returned expressing concerns that the minority students they observed seemed isolated from the mainstream of the student body. In my experience, this simply doesn't happen at the earlier levels. When children are younger, prejudices that have already been formed are more easily stripped away, and when they have not been formed, they are unlikely to emerge. It is a responsibility of any junior boarding school to incorporate a multicultural student body that allows children to experience a range of ethnic and racial differences.

Most junior boarding schools have understood the value of bringing together socio-economic extremes, but the participation of the middle group has led to a new phenomenon. Perhaps it is because my institution has a relatively modest physical plant that we are experiencing increasing admission interest from middle income families rather than those seeking an elitist environment for their children. Although this has put a strain on financial aid budgets of most junior schools, it has resulted in a very healthy acceptance of a child for his individual talents. One of the strengths of a boarding school is its ability to put everyone on a level socio-economic footing on which people must earn respect for their talents rather than their financial wherewithal. Our younger students receive $3 a week in allowance and the older ones $5. When weekend events are offered that require additional spending, we take considerable time discussing the importance of exercising financial restraint. At the secondary level, boarding students are generally given freer reign to spend, and in some schools credit cards are given to the students for that purpose. I would venture to say that a boarding student in a conscientiously-designed junior program will gain a greater sense of financial responsibility than in a family setting where parents are on hand to support a child's every whim. A student will generally be better positioned to make mature decisions regarding finances when he enters secondary school.

Convincing parents of the practicality of boarding schools is sometimes easier than convincing their children. For some prospective students, boarding represents an opportunity to gain independence and share 24 hours a day with peers, while for others it represents being thrust out of the home into a new, very frightening environment where they will encounter many unknowns. In actuality, the boarding experience lies somewhere in between. Being honest with a prospective student requires striking a balance between the pros and cons of boarding during the interview process. Certainly it is important to generate interest by highlighting the activities that can be enjoyed, but it is equally important to identify frustrations that accompany community living. A good boarding experience should not emulate summer camp; instead, it should mirror all the hardships and frustrations that would be encountered at home. It is unrealistic and even unhealthy to live a life devoid of hardships; therefore, it is imperative that the boarding experience include some obstacles that will be burdensome and help develop sound character. In many situations those tasks that would seem unpalatable and cause friction at home become much easier for a child to accept in a boarding environment. A case in point is the way a child endures the task of attacking homework at boarding school. When dinner ends at 6:45 and the evening study hall commences, instead of feeling that he is the only person in the world that must be forced to confront a mountain of homework, the boarding student sees that peers are faced with the same tasks. This makes studying much less of a chore.

The flip side of the independence gained is the restrictions and structure attendant to students in a boarding community. When study hall ends in the evening and phone calls need to be placed to parents, limitations must be set for the frequency of calls and length of conversation. By being part of the group, one must, like it or not, learn that freedoms previously taken for granted no longer exist. The lights-out policy presents another interesting study. In my own home, there has never been any set procedure regarding bedtimes. My three children have demonstrated individual sleep requirements that can dictate when they will retire each evening. In a dormitory it would be foolhardy to allow much flexibility in bedtime; therefore, keeping very precise hours for lights out is essential. This can seem burdensome for those who are used to "calling the shots" at home or have patterns that require fewer hours of sleep. Even such mundane exercises as showering require restrictions in a small dormitory with limited shower facilities. Herding people through the showering process takes time and patience and on occasion necessitates a scheduling pattern that poses an inconvenience. At meals, flexibility once again becomes impractical. When a meal begins everyone must be present, and if a pattern of tardiness occurs, consequences must be put in place. In our school, this most often will be in the form of early bedtime.

As limitations are instituted for these young boarders, they sometimes refuse to conform to expectations without a degree of rebellion. It requires a certain personality to deal with a dorm full of pre-adolescents testing the limits. Finding good people who want to devote themselves to dorm-parenting is not an easy task. In interviewing candidates who will serve as both teacher and dorm parent for children who are as young as 10 or 11 years old, I have to make our school's objectives perfectly clear. The work in the dormitory must always take precedence over coaching or teaching responsibilities. If a child is in distress, responding to him cannot be delayed even if there is a class preparation needed for the next day. Balancing the needs of children can present a serious dilemma for a serious young teachers who set high standards for themselves in the classroom.

Likewise, a teacher with family has decisions to make. What priority is placed upon a person's privacy and family life when balanced against the responsibilities of serving as a dormitory parent? Should a teacher sacrifice the peace and tranquility of his own relationship with spouse and children to make the dormitory the warm, loving enclave that can nurture young boarding students devoid of daily family contact? These are never easy questions, and in a junior boarding school structure it is beneficial to give time off to dorm faculty because when they are on duty, they are truly "on." The young age of the junior boarder implies that a firmer structure be in place and this translates into an intense working environment. At the secondary level the dorm parent's responsibility is to be a presence, monitoring students and being available when a crisis occurs. At younger levels a good boarding parent must stand ready to join in and participate in any given activity, whether it be a hike up a mountainside, a game of capture-the-flag or a trip to the movies. The intensity of serving as a constant role model and consistently setting limits for young boarders puts a premium on patience and imagination. For this reason all our school's dormitory parents work in teams that alternate being on-duty weekday nights and weekends.

An alternative to the boarding couple with family is the young, eager boarding faculty member who has recently graduated from college. Invariably this individual has idealistic aspirations of working and molding young children. Regardless of how black the picture is painted for these prospective teachers, the on-the-job realities are a shock to their systems. For a person who has had total independence and freedom in college to suddenly be saddled with a dormitory responsibility is a tremendous jolt, and only a certain personality can make the transition smoothly. Resumes must include significant interaction with children; otherwise, the achievements listed are virtually meaningless. The interview is critical, and if a person is concerned about protecting his private life, it is a "red flag." I'll often ask prospective boarding parents how they might feel about spending the night comforting a child who is throwing up into a toilet bowl and then facing classes the next day. This is the acid test of a good young boarding parent. I look for people who have what I consider a social worker make-up. For young single dormitory parents I also look for one who will be able to fill the role of a big brother or sister for younger people. The ideal combination for dormitory parents is a young, but very mature, single person and an older couple, with or without children. The compatibility of these two units must be extraordinarily strong because they may be "played off" against each other in the same manner that children "split" two biological parents. A child who has experienced divorce or separation at home is likely to have mastered the art of working one parent against the other.

As soon as a student has settled into a dormitory, he will, consciously or subconsciously, begin the process of comparing his dorm parents. Generally he will feel a greater chemistry with one than the other and will form a closer bond as a result. He will sometimes recognize vulnerability in a dorm parent which can be perceived as a sign of weakness. For this reason, at our school we structure faculty working schedules so that all dormitory parents work together during the first two weekends each fall. In this way they can synchronize their responses as well as possible and establish a consistency that will serve the children well during the year. While individual styles of dorm-parenting are encouraged, junior boarding students thrive on continuity, and dorm parents must be unified in the values they present to their charges.

Although secondary boarding schools espouse teaching values to students, it is the junior boarding school where values are ingrained much more deliberately. A good junior boarding school should have regular courses in human sexuality and substance abuse, but it is the responsibility of the boarding system to monitor the safety of the students. Direct supervision is essential in ensuring a drug-free, sexually safe environment, and open communication between students and dorm parents is imperative. The dorm parents must not only serve as impeccable role models, but must also establish the rapport and trust that encourages open communication with students. In a coeducational setting such as Bement's, it is important to establish an adult presence at all times and eliminate opportunities for children to experiment with sex. Yes, dances are occasionally scheduled and relationships between boys and girls are expected to develop, but the responsibility for protecting students must be recognized as a priority. Therefore, at our school hand-holding between buildings is permitted and social opportunities are frequently scheduled. The boys are, however, dismissed separately from study hall because the walk back to the dormitory is long and dark. Under no circumstances are the girls and boys allowed to be alone together in a dormitory. All of these precautions are taken to delay sexual experimentation. In a junior boarding school it is not good enough to provide condoms with the premise that sexual intercourse is inevitable. It is our responsibility to monitor coed interaction and, therefore, minimize the risks that are associated with active sexual behavior. All of this is done knowing that surveys find that 36 percent of junior high school girls have had sexual intercourse. Although going against the flow of teenage habits is difficult, it helps delay these decisions for young adolescents until a time when they can make a more mature decision. The prevailing teenage attitude towards substance abuse is similar and, therefore, the structures imposed must be consistently tight. A good junior boarding school has this obligation to both its students and their families.

There clearly are an intimidating set of obstacles which any school encounters in setting up a boarding environment in which children can be safe and happy. Only the most responsible program with mature and committed leadership will work well. Soliciting parental support is particularly critical if a child is to succeed in adjusting to a junior boarding environment. Invariably the parent lacking rapport with or strong guidelines for his child becomes an authority on child-rearing when his child enters a boarding setting. Away at school when the child balks about restrictions, the parent is ultimately torn between supporting school policy and "feeding the fuel" of discontent. Only the strong conviction and the united stance of dorm parent and biological parent can ensure a clear statement that a person can embrace. It requires confidence for a parent to tell a petulant child that an unpopular dorm parent decision is surely in his best interest. Only with this support does a school have the leverage to create a consistent, structured environment in which a child can blossom personally and academically.

While it is easy to focus on the visible pitfalls of a junior boarding education, the advantages are often intangible. If the right combination of dorm parents is in place, and there is a good working relationship between parent and dorm parent, an optimum environment can evolve. There are significant opportunities for children to gain independence by being placed in an environment outside the family realm. In addition, the consistency that results from a controlled boarding environment can help the student develop study habits that will continue to serve the child well in secondary school and beyond. In a rapidly changing world, parents find that limits are increasingly difficult to establish for youngsters, particularly when parents have a very full agenda of their own. For these people in particular, the junior boarding school can serve an important function.

In a society in which children spend a disproportionate amount of time looking for action at the mall or on the street corner, a well-conceived junior boarding program can offer a healthy and often wholesome alternative. There is a place in our educational system for junior boarding schools if one is able to get beyond the emotional concerns conjured up by the concept.

15

Therapeutic Mentoring: Beyond Teaching And Therapy

By Henry T. Radda, Ph.D.
Dean of Students
The John Dewey Academy
Great Barrington, Massachusetts

The alienated adolescent, in specific, needs therapeutic mentoring. This chapter delineates the clinical experience of the teachers and therapists at The John Dewey Academy, a residential college preparatory therapeutic high school. The traditional boundaries of clinical and academic staff have been modified. We utilize the concept of mentor to humanize the teaching and therapeutic work that is done with these adolescents. Mentoring is a necessary condition to help these adolescents who have parents and professionals flaunting their authority. A developmental approach is described for cultivating a therapeutic mentoring relationship.

Therapeutic Mentoring: Beyond Teaching And Therapy

> The good teacher educates by his speech and by his silence, in the hours of teaching and in the recesses, in casual conversation, through his mere existence, only he must be a really exciting man and he must be really present to his pupils: he educates through contact.
>
> (Buber, 1967)

The mentor lives by the principles that Buber elucidates. The first expectation of the mentor is personal involvement. The relationship between Anne Sullivan and Helen Keller (Lash, 1980) is a good example; in it we see a wholly personal involvement in the way Anne educates Helen. Anne not only had to dedicate herself in matters scholastic, but she needed to teach Helen manners, values and attitudes. Personal involvement is crucial. Bettelheim (1974) describes how the personal involvement of the staff is a necessity and a requirement for working in the school he developed. Barr (1971) endorses this involvement and refutes programmed and mechanized teaching precisely because of the lack of human contact. He says, "These devices lack wonderment, respect, and love." There is no question that, in working with a population of alienated adolescents, the worst possible solution is to adopt a cold, detached and analytical stance. Alienated students need to be educated by mentors who are willing to risk being hurt by becoming personally involved.

Ethel, previously hospitalized for attempted suicide, depressions and self-destructive behavior came to our school at 13. To risk, to care, to become involved with her could be emotionally draining—it was. Each time we met to do math, her first words were, "I can't." She disliked math because it reinforced her feeling of stupidity. In each class we struggled together through the examples. Even after completing a problem correctly she would utter, "I can't!" Her self-defeatist attitude pervaded academics, and her social interactions permeated her being. Therapeutic interactions were similar to the academic ones. I found real steps of accomplishment and encouragement, found positive thoughts and highlighted them, and used humor whenever possible to push her out of her abyss.

Ethel flourished academically after a year of persistence from her, myself and the other staff. New teachers, who did not know her during the first year, couldn't believe she was ever a poor student. The new English teacher praised her merits in every other staff meeting. It was welcome news. Emotionally, the battle took longer with many ups and downs, wins and losses. The role of mentor calls for an involvement which creates opportunity for pain when the person fails and triumph when the person succeeds.

The mentor "educates through contact." He or she needs to be able to empathize with the adolescent. The importance of empathy is evidenced in counseling by Truax and Carkhuff (1967) and in teaching by Rogers (1969). Shultz (1967) describes empathy; "We may grasp the other's experience with the same perceptual intention that we grasp a thing or event presented to us." Moustakes (1981) describes how the therapist makes use of his/her experiences internally to empathize and approximate the position of the child. The principle of empathy is a process because the mentor continually must consider the needs and abilities of the mentee. This distinguishes empathy from sympathy. The mentor must empathize, but then be able to demonstrate, suggest, or demand that the mentee move forward. The point of empathy is not to get stuck with the mentee but to help the mentee gather all of his/her resources towards growth. Daloz (1983) points out:

> Although he is supportive, a mentor is by no means mindlessly sanguine. In place of certainties, we prod, cajole, urge. Indeed, the kind

of challenge that good teachers have to offer is the prospect of the journey itself because we have been there and our charges have not.

It would have been easy to just sympathize with Ethel on how terrible things had been for her. She had been neglected, abused, scarred for life in an accident and endured innumerable other misfortunes. It was not fair. There was no simple solution. She would have to work academically and emotionally. I had to convey to her that I understood where she came from; however, in no way did I have to agree with her negativistic view of the future based on her past. At times. I felt like quitting, saying, "You're right, people will hurt you, you will fail again and make mistakes, it is difficult." My job however was to push her beyond that by making her look at her accomplishments, her victories and her ability to survive what many would not.

The mentor needs to establish his or her own expertness in helping others. This can be done in various ways, but the student must believe in the ability of the mentor to help. Professionals must demonstrate that they can identify the games adolescents play. These kids despise teachers and therapists who allow them continually to avoid reality, that is, the limits and consequences of their behavior. These alienated adolescents have little internal structure. They have turned off their consciousness with chemicals or defense mechanisms. Masterson (1981) describes how the therapist must patiently, consistently confront the adolescent with reality, yet, through behavior, demonstrates the value of trust in the relationship. Adolescents respect the teacher and therapist who calls their games and bluffs. They can feel safe with such a person—one who has the awareness, experience and courage to be honest and forthright with them. To them the world lacks coherence because they have been able to manipulate it, often to their own detriment. The mentor must demonstrate that he or she has the ability to help them by knowing them, not their projections of defense, but the person they are inside. The mentor then has legitimacy to them.

Harvey had come for one interview at our school. Through his telling of stories of how he was, his street experience, and acting provocatively, he expected us to be impressed and/or intimidated. We acted nonchalantly and continued to question him about the pain he must feel to have to act so tough and strong. We made it clear that if he were really that "bad," that far gone, that The John Dewey Academy would be the wrong place for him. I told him I could refer him to another program where there would be criminals, heroin addicts and murderers. When I said this matter-of-factly, Harvey knew I was serious. He recognized the staff was firm and experienced and so realized that it would be in his best interest to change.

Harvey's game was brinkmanship. The mentor must know how far to push the adolescent and when to give another alternative so as not to create a destructive situation. Ninety-five percent of the adolescents we interview do not test or exceed the limits, once they respect not only the knowledge and experience of the staff but also their humanity.

A powerful tool of the mentor is to demonstrate expertness in the reputation he/she has with the student. When an adolescent receives a positive report about a staff member from a peer, it is useful. In our intake interviews with perspective applicants, students sit in and give tours on which they can talk candidly. It is amazing that when some return from their tours, they realize that the staff is knowledgeable and will not be manipulated.

The personal and professional attainments of the mentor are important to the student. They demonstrate the mentor's implementation of his/her talent(s). The mentor, by virtue of his or her accomplishments and demonstration that he or she can help other adolescents, gives the individual a sense of hope. The mentor has a charisma, which is important in the early stages of the adolescents struggle to grow. (Radda, 1988)

The next guiding principle described by Levinson (1978) is "finding the DREAM." Through interviewing, the mentor searches with questions to see if the mentee has lost, given up on, or destroyed the DREAM. The mentor asks, "Did you ever have any hope, any direction, any goal that really mattered to you?" It is crucial and demands much skill, especially with an alienated, negativistic or passive adolescent, to create the condition, to dare to DREAM. The mentor's expertise will be necessary to help the adolescent identify a path and define the necessary changes to secure the DREAM. The DREAM is the adolescent's hope that has been buried or temporarily lost.

Encouraging and giving hope are essential, especially in regard to alienated adolescents. Scotland (1969) describes the crucial ingredient in therapy of hope. Radda (1988) describes the importance of giving hope to the alienated adolescents in believing in his or her DREAM. These adolescents, although gifted, doubt themselves and need someone who believes in them. It will take much experience for them to believe in themselves once again or for the first time. Helen Keller (1954) describes the importance of the first spark of hope:

> Once I knew the depth where no hope was and darkness lay on the face of all things. Then love came and set my soul free. Once I fretted and beat myself against the wall that shut me in. My life was without a past or future, and death a consummation devoutly to be wished. But a little word from the fingers of another fell into my hands that clutched at emptiness, and my heart leaped up with the rapture of living. I do not know the meaning of the darkness, but I have learned the overcoming of it.

These adolescents need a mentor who will encourage them through their struggle. Hardeman (1985) underscores this when he explains that "some outstanding scientists and engineers have reported initially low self-esteem, but stressed the influence of a role model who provided encouragement."

Modeling is described by Baudura (1977) as one of the most powerful methods of psychological change. Levinson (1978), Jones (1982), and Humm & Reissman (1988) describe the mentor as a role model. Bratter, Bratter & Radda (1986) have further discussed the importance of the responsible role model in the therapeutic high school. Personal qualities are viewed as necessary conditions for working with these adolescents. The mentor is often scrutinized by the student: how he/she acts, lives, grows or stagnates; how he/she is responsible. The student is sensitive to hypocrisy as described by Bratter (1987). The student searches for someone to believe in but will not accept falsehood. He or she has been burned before. The responsible role model has to be willing to confront doubt and demonstrate responsibility. Glasser (1965) describes the importance of the therapist demonstrating his or her responsibility in the face of difficulty. The mentor must model belief and dedication to personal and academic excellence.

Recently, one of the graduates, who is now a senior at Williams College, related an experience that was important to him while he attended our school. He was having difficulty studying. I suggested he come upstairs and study with me. At the time I was reading *Fundamentals of Neuropsychopharmacology*, not easy material. I related to him that reading and understanding the material was laborious and could require up to five minutes a page. I read him some of the material and he agreed it was cumbersome and overly scientific, not written for the layman. He found the experience of studying with me and watching me struggle through difficult material helped motivate him. To this day he says when he has trouble studying he remembers me reading him what they use to do to the rats brains in the blender to determine different level of neurotransmitter.

The mentor inspires learning. The quest for knowledge is apparent in the mentor. The student is inspired by the mentor to wonder, question, investigate and learn. The mentor shows the relevance of learning first by modeling and second by explaining. The student may have lost reason or belief in education, as described by Bratter (1985). But the mentor can help the student see the power and the rejuvenation that can come from knowledge.

The mentor has a powerful tool to use judicious self-disclosure. Jourard (1958), Weiner (1983) and Simon (1988) describe the uses of self-disclosure. The mentor can use his or her own resolved conflicts or problems to demonstrate hope and ability to overcome difficulties. The student can sense that the mentor knows what to do. Bratter (1984) describes the adult's revisiting of his or her own adolescence to understand the adolescent, and to communicate that understanding. The therapist, by using him or herself, reveals humanness and accessibility. Glasser (1965) describes the use of disclosure to demonstrate the understanding that responsible behavior may be difficult but required.

The therapist must be sure to disclose for the good of the mentee. Lasmmert (1986) reiterates that the responsible therapist must be aware of his or her own reasons for self-disclosing. In the beginning, disclosure is used to demonstrate understanding of the student's position, and knowledge and ability to transcend the present position. The mentor uses self-disclosure to model appropriate successful behavior and attitudes. The mentoring relationship calls for a very personal, intimate relationship where disclosure inevitably occurs. The mentor must therefore be aware and open to the impact of disclosures verbally and behaviorally.

The expectations of the mentor are high. Jones (1982) describes mentors as "demanding much of their proteges." The mentor must help the mentee with whom he has empathized to move forward. The mentor is willing to sustain the anger, rage, hurt, loneliness, alienation of the adolescent and still demand growth and improvement. Bratter (1985) describes how many have already given up on these youth. The mentor must be willing to demonstrate through persistent intervention the sincere belief that more responsible behavior is expected. Only if expectations continue to step ahead will the student grow, until the adolescent again starts to believe in him or herself.

The mentor relationship is dynamic. It changes with time in terms of power. The mentee originally gains much power from the persona of the mentor: knowledge, skills, integrity, charisma, and experience. Over time the mentor relinquishes authority and power when the adolescent demonstrates a competence to take control of behavior. This change of authority and power are necessary for the relationship to remain healthy as described by Radda (1990). Ethel's mentor must be willing and able to give the adolescent room to grow on her own. Ethel is still concerned and would protest any self-destructive behavior, however, the goal is towards self-respect, accountability and responsibility. This is important for one who had no longer even trusted him or herself. The adolescent recognizes that the mentor trusts him more and offers opinion less often, waiting for the adolescent to make more moves on his own.

In conclusion, the mentor must be personally involved, be empathetic not sympathetic, demonstrate charisma and expertness, help the adolescent find his DREAM, encourage and give hope to that DREAM, judiciously self-disclose, model responsible behavior, demand the best from the protege and renegotiate the relationship when the adolescent demands a new maturity.

Bibliography

Aguiliar-Gaxiola, S. (1984). "The Role of Mentors in the Lives of Graduate Students." Paper presented at the Annual Meeting of the American Educational Research Association, New Orleans, La., April 23-27, 1984.

Alleman, E., J. Cochran, J. Doverspike, & I. Newman, (1984). "Enriching Mentoring Relationships." *The Personal and Guidance Journal.* Feb. 1984, vol. 62, pp. 329-332.

Bandura, A. (1977). *Social Learning Theory.* Englewood Cliffs, N.J.: Prentice Hall.

Barr, D. (1971). *Who Pushed Humpty Dumpty? Dilemmas in American Educations Today.* New York: Atheneum.

Bettleim, B. (1974). *A Home for the Heart.* New York: Alfred A. Knopf.

Bratter, T.E., E.P. Bratter, L.J. Greenfield, H.T. Radda "The Evolution of The Responsible Role Model: Its Relevance to the Pedagogical Relationship and to Dewey's Educational Thought." in A. Compora & E. Nedelkopf (eds.), *The Proceedings of the 9th World Conference of Therapeutic Communities*. San Francisco: Abacus Printing, 1986, pp. 292-298.

Bratter, T.E., B.I. Bratter & H.T. Radda, "The John Dewey Academy: A Residential Therapeutic High School." *Journal of Substance Abuse Treatment*. 1986 (3), pp. 53-58.

Daloz, L.A. (1983). "Mentors: Teachers Who Make a Difference." *Change*. Sept. 1983, vol 15, pp. 24-27.

Delisle, J.R. (1986). "Death With Honors: Suicide Among Gifted Adolescents." *Journal of Counseling and Development*. May 1986. vol 64(9), pp. 558-560.

Edlind, E. P. & P. A. Hanensly, (1985). "Gifts of Mentorship." *Gifted Child Quarterly*. Spring 1985, vol. 29(2), pp. 55-60.

Gerstein, M. (1985). "Mentoring: An Age Old Practice in a Knowledge -Based Society." *Journal of Counseling & Development*. Oct. 1985, vol. 64(2), pp.156-157.

Glasser, W. (1965). *Reality Therapy*. New York: Harper and Row.

Humm, A. & F. Riessman (1988), "Peer Mentoring: An Anti-Drop-Out Strategy." In N. S. Giddan(ed.), *Community and Social Support for College Students*. Toledo OH.: Charles C. Thomas. pp. 177-190.

Hardeman, C.H. (1985). "The Quest for Excellence/Pupil Self-Esteem." *In: Invited Papers: Elementary/Secondary Education Data Redesign Project*. Oct. 1985, pp. 18-26.

"Instruction, and Mentoring Functions with Academically Deficient College Freshman." *Journal of Educations Research*. Jan-Fed. 1977, vol. 70(3), pp. 142-147.

Jourard, S.M. (1985). *Personal Adjustment*. Toronto: Macmillan.

Kaiser, C.F. & D.J. Berndt. (1985). "Predictors of Loneliness in the Gifted Adolescent. *Gifted Child Quarterly*. Spring 1985, vol. 29(2), pp 74-77.

Keller, H. (1954) *The Story of My Life*. New York: Doubleday.

Kolodny, R.C., N.J. Kolodny, T.E. Bratter, & C. Deep. *How to Survive Your Adolescent's Adolescence*. Boston: Little Brown.

Lasmmert, M. (1986). "Experience as Knowing: Utilizing Therapist Self Awareness." *Social Casework: The Journal of Contemporary Social Work*. June 1986, pp. 369-376.

Lash, J.P. (1980) *Helen and Teacher*. London: Penguin.

Levinson, D.J. (1979). *The Seasons of a Man's Life*. New York: A.A. Knopf.

Levinson, D.J. (1978). "Growing Up With The Dream." *Psychology Today*. Jan. 1978, vol. 12, pp. 20-89.

Masterson, J. F. (1981). *The Narcissistic and Borderline Disorders*. New York: Brunner/Mazel Inc.

Moustakes, C. (1981). *Rhythms, Rituals and Relationships*. Detroit, MI.: Harlo Press.

Philips-Jones, L. (1982). *Mentors and Proteges*. New York: Arbor.

Obler, M., K. Francis, & R. Wishengrad (1977). "Combination of traditional Counseling," Radda, H.T. "Extending the Therapeutic Alliance: Mentorship." *The Journal of Reality Therapy*. Fall 1988.

Radda, H.T. *Extending the Therapeutic Relationship: A Psychotherapeutic Treatment Model For Bright, Alienated, Acting-Out Adolescents*. Doctoral Dissertation, 1990.

Rogers, C. (1969). *Freedom to Learn*. "Gifted Adolescents as Co-learners in Mentorships." *Journal for the Education of the Gifted*. Vol. VIII(2), 1985, pp. 127-132.

Schockett, M. & M. Haring-Hidore. (1985). "Factor Analytic Support for Psychosocial and Vocational Mentoring Functions." *Psychological Reports*, July, 1985, vol. 57, pp. 627-630.

Schoenfield, W. "The Psychotherapist as Friend" in A. Bassin, T.E. Bratter & R.L. Rachin (eds.), *The Reality Therapy Reader*, New York: Harper & Row, 1976, pp. 119-132.

Shultz, A. (1967). *The Phenomenology of the Social World*. Evanstron, IL.: Northwestern University Press.

Scotland, E. (1969). *The Psychology of Hope*. San Francisco: Jossey-Bass Inc.

Simon, J.C. (1988). "Criteria for Therapist Self Disclosure." *American Journal of Psychotherapy*. July 1988, vol. XLII(3), pp. 404-415.

Truax C. & Carkhuff R. (1967). *Toward Effective Counseling and Psychotherapy: Training and Practice*. Chicago: Aldine Publishing.

Weiner, M.F. (1983). *Therapist Disclosure: The Use Of Self in Psychotherapy*. (2nd. ed.). Baltimore: University Park Press.

16

Gender in the Dorm

by Sarah Unsworth Jordan
Dublin School
Dublin, New Hampshire

You're on campus patrol, "walkabout," on a Friday night. None of the students seem to be in the dorm, but you take a walk down the corridor to check. There is an odor of aftershave, orange peels and Ben Gay; someone also has been cooking popcorn recently. The rooms are in moderate disarray, but the bathroom is neat except for a few paper towels lying by the wastebasket. On the walls there are pictures of heavy metal rock stars, girls in bathing suits, and men skiing. There is a hole in the wall by the outside door.

In the next dorm, no one is at home either. Someone has made popcorn here, too. The rooms are generally neater, but the bathroom is draped with underwear and pantyhose and there are many brushes around the sink. On the bathroom door there is a poster of a baby playing with a roll of toilet paper. In some of the rooms are pictures of muscular men in bathing suits, but there are also stuffed animals on some of the beds. A hand-lettered sign near the door explains at some length why there will be a dorm-cleaning and inspection tonight; it is signed by the dorm proctor.

Whatever else boarding school faculty may say about dormitory life, most of us agree that boys' dorms and girls' dorms are different. The differences begin with decor, but they are far more significant than that. The "gender gap" extends to dormitory organization and problems and to faculty perceptions of where the challenges and satisfactions lie in working with one sex or the other. Our effectiveness as dorm parents depends to a certain extent on our willingness to acknowledge these gender differences and to work with them, rather than bemoaning or ignoring them.

Conflict and Intimacy

One way to gain insight into gender issues in the dorm is to look at the kinds of problems which dorm parents commonly report as particular to boys' dorms and girls' dorms. The most obvious differences center around the way each gender tends to deal with conflict. Less often discussed, but equally significant, is the difference in the way that boys and girls deal with emotional intimacy; this also contributes to the differences between girls' and boys' dormitories.

Conflict in a boys' dorm is usually easy to spot. A hole appears in the bathroom wall; a fistfight breaks out in the commons; a shouting match is heard down the hall. You follow the trail of physical evidence until you find the combatants, you get some eyewitness accounts, you sit down with everybody involved, and you try to talk it out. The presenting issue will often involve territory and rights: the right to play one's music at 100 decibels versus the right to have peace and quiet in the next room; who gets to watch what on the dorm television; whether or not someone had permission to borrow someone else's walkman, bicycle, compact disc. There may well be other issues below the surface, but you may never hear about these unless you ask very specific questions. Chronic personality conflicts, if they emerge, may result in a pattern of small scuffles and persistent verbal baiting, with physical strength becoming the deciding factor. Physical harassment can (and should) be dealt with through the disciplinary system. Emotional abuse among peers is more difficult to spot in a boys' dorm, since boys in our culture usually feel it is "uncool" to complain about being bullied by other boys; they should be able to handle it themselves, they believe. But hurt feelings can simmer in a boys' dorm, just as they do in a girls' dorm, until resentments erupt into violence.

In a girls' dorm, conflict is a little more complicated to deal with: the holes appear not in the walls, but in the fabric of relationships in the dorm community; the issues revolve around rights and territory, but the territory extends into the psychological sphere. Offense can be given and taken in more subtle ways than in a boys dorm. As one female student remarked to me, "It's done with words, yes, but it doesn't even take words—you can tell somebody what you think about them with just body language." Moderating disputes and intervening in personality conflicts is correspondingly complex for the dorm parent in a girls' dormitory. Both male and female faculty remark that conflict in girls' dorms is harder to resolve, in part because of the denial that there is real conflict. As one of my male colleagues put it, "Girls put on that bright, rosy face. . . . They feel they should be accepting of other people and so they think about it (conflict) more and carry it around inside." A girl in the same faculty member's dorm added her own insight into that dynamic: "Ten minutes after you've had a fight with someone, you usually feel guilty about it," she said. "So, you go find the other person and make it up with her—whether or not you've really solved the problem."

On the other hand, boarding faculty remark on how much more girls tend to support each other emotionally, whether on the sports team or in the dormitory. The same sensitivity to nuance which renders conflict so complicated becomes an asset when directed toward the understanding of another's heartache; most girls comprehend feelings of vulnerability all too well. Both male and female faculty can call upon this strength of female students as they help them to resolve conflicts in the dormitory. Often, girls need to "check out" verbally the perceived meaning of nonverbal signals. A look or touch which one girl thinks of as harmless teasing, another girl may take as hostility or as an invasion of privacy. Yet we tell females in our culture that it is "bitchy" to confront someone else about an affront to our self-esteem. So, girls perceive it as safer to nurse a misunderstanding than to tell other girls—or boys—when they have done something offensive. Faculty can provide for girls a safe forum for airing anger and hurt feelings. They can encourage girls to be direct and make sure that they are not penalized for speaking their minds. After the negative feelings are articulated honestly, the instinct for social harmony can come back into play in a more healthy way.

Girls perceive relationships and the whole process of growing up as requiring discussion, analysis, evaluation. In an anonymous survey of boarding students at Dublin School, girls said, almost without exception, that they felt a need for an older female with whom they could talk about "girl stuff"—a term which appeared to encompass everything from questions about the menstrual cycle to bafflement over the interactions they had with boys. Male faculty were not seen as appropriate guides in these matters, although almost all the girls surveyed mentioned that they felt having a "father figure" in the dorm created a "balance" and a more family-like atmosphere. Girls are at risk for pregnancy as soon as they become sexually active, and the female reproductive tract is particularly vulnerable to sexually transmitted diseases. If only for these health reasons, it really is imperative that girls have access to at least one female dorm parent who is knowledgeable and comfortable about discussing these issues. A school nurse also may be available for this task; but often the questions surface more easily in the intimacy of the dorm setting than during an "official" visit to the health services.

Girls, more than boys, tend to be conscious of the dorm as a functioning social unit, and critique it on the basis of how much community is experienced there. At Dublin, one 9th-grade girl related with delight the memory of an evening when "the whole dorm was squeezed into the common room, just watching TV together and making jokes about the commercials, and everyone was getting along really well." That moment of physical and emotional community, she remembered as "one of the high points of my year in the dorm." That same student remarked that the basic social structure of the dorm revolved around roommate relationships, which tended to be close. "You don't talk to everybody in the dorm about your bad day," she said, "but I can say anything to my roommate. We can get mad at each other, too. But we always talk it out afterwards, when we've cooled down."

Boys' dormitories do not come by emotional closeness so readily. Boys are less likely to discuss their emotional state with their male peers, particularly if that involves voicing feelings like homesickness, confusion, or grief over the loss of a relationship. Many boys still feel that they "lose face" by revealing their vulnerabilities. Some of the boys I surveyed at Dublin talked about the need for an older male with whom they could discuss "guy stuff" but this term seemed more limited to questions about sexuality and hygiene. A couple of boys remarked specifically that they felt more comfortable discussing emotional problems with a woman. On the other hand, several boys who lived in a dormitory with single male dorm parents talked about the satisfactions of having common activities and interests they could share with their resident faculty. They seemed to doubt that a female—or for that matter, a married male resident faculty member—could become close to the dorm members without sharing these interests—specifically sports. Social cohesiveness in a boys' dorm tends to revolve around common activities, whereas in a girls' dorm the goal of the activity is often to provide an opportunity to talk about feelings. Dorm parents in a boys' dorm need to make sure their students know they are available for discussion of the interpersonal dynamics of the dorm. They can provide a safe opportunity for the airing of feelings of failure, loneliness and sadness, feelings of which our culture tells boys to be ashamed. It should be okay to cry in the presence of your dorm parent, even if you are an adolescent male. Feelings of grief or inadequacy do not have to be "fixed" right away. Sometimes it is more important simply to experience them in the presence of a supportive adult.

See How They Grow
The above observations are anecdotal rather than scientific. They are based on my own experiences as a dorm parent in both boys' and girls' dormitories over a period of about ten years, and on many conversations with my colleagues in the schools where I have worked. But they are also in line with the theories of Carol Gilligan, set forth in her landmark book, *In a Different Voice*, a work which has had a great impact on the way I have come to view gender differences. Gilligan's most important contribution to the understanding of gender issues has been her reframing of perceptions which others have verified through social research. Gilligan is particularly skillful at articulating the ways in which we often perceive female behavior as deviant rather than simply different from male behavior. She also has some very relevant points to make about the ways males and females handle conflict and intimacy.

Gilligan begins by citing the work of Nancy Chodorow and of Janet Lever. Chodorow, writing during the 70s, described the development of gender identity as involving different tasks for girls and boys. Girls, she says, identify as female by identifying with their mothers, usually the primary childcare provider, while boys gain their gender identity by differentiating themselves from their female care providers. According to Chodorow, girls experience themselves as "more continuous with" the external world because their primary experience of who they are involves the experience of being like their mothers. Boys, on the other hand, experience themselves as different from their mothers and thus, as more distinct from the world they live in. So, adds Gilligan, we shouldn't be surprised that "male gender identity is threatened by intimacy while female gender identity is threatened by separation. Thus, males tend to have difficulty with relationships while females tend to have problems with individuation." Gilligan ties this into the observations of Janet Lever, who studied elementary school students in 1976. Lever noted the differences in the ways that male and female students played games during recess and after school. She remarked that boys' games, although more competitive, lasted longer than girls' games "because, when disputes arose in the course of a game, boys were able to resolve the disputes more effectively than girls." While boys actually seemed to enjoy the legal disputes over rules and cheating, girls ended their games rather than jeopardize their relationships with the other players by quarreling. A "legal resolution" to disputes was seen by girls as potentially hurting some players in order to continue the activity; this was unacceptable.

The above synopsis is simplified; Gilligan cites many prominent social scientists in her discussion of adolescent and adult moral development. But, simply put, her conclusion is that human psychic development, as it has been described by psychologists since Freud, is based on a male model. The hallmark of maturity, according to this model, is autonomy; but women, says Gilligan, mature differently. For women, knowing oneself is inextricably tied to understanding one's interdependency with other people. Women's development process links moral maturity to "the understanding of responsibility and relationships," while men's psychological development leads to their viewing of morality as tied to "the understanding of rights and rules."

If Gilligan's thesis is valid, then we can expect to see these differences in male and female identity affecting the way we work, play, and the things we argue about. And that, in my experience, is the case. I never understood until I returned to full-time professional work, how deep the conflict would be between my right to fulfill myself in my career and my responsibility to fulfill my role as a mother and spouse. It is a conflict of which I am aware every day of my working life. Yet my husband, a sensitive and nurturing father, does not experience that conflict with the same intensity; nor do most of the men I work with. I have seen, time and again, similar conflicts arise in the lives of my female friends: an inability to easily put aside the quarrel that arose in the dorm, the disagreement with the boyfriend, and get down to work on their assignments; a tendency to put the nurturing of relationships first, whether or not that is wise in terms of their academic success or involvement in the disciplinary system. That is not to say that boys are not distracted by their emotional involvements and problems; obviously, they are. But boys are less able to articulate the reasons for their distraction, whereas girls can often tell you in painful detail exactly why they are feeling and acting so miserable. I believe that for boys, escape from emotional turmoil into autonomous activity is experienced as legitimate and good; while for girls, there remains a nagging sense of unfinished business as long as the inter-personal conflicts remain unresolved.

The Dorm Parent's Challenge

If we accept the proposition that boys and girls operate differently because they arrive at adolescence with different agendas, then what are the challenges for dorm parents—particularly for dorm parents of the opposite sex from the students they are supervising? Does age and marital status make a difference in faculty relations with students in the dorm? And what are some of the pitfalls that faculty need to avoid in supervising girls' dorms and boys' dorms? To these more practical questions I want to turn my attention for the rest of this chapter.

A primary challenge for the dorm parent is to be sensitive to gender differences and the issues that arise from these. Whether we are parenting students of the same sex or of the opposite sex, this should mean examining our own stereotypes about male and female behavior. This is an uncomfortable process; but as teachers, we have a commitment to continue our own learning, and this includes, in my view, learning about our own emotional patterns and prejudices. Over and over again, I've found that it was exactly the student who got under my skin the most who ended up teaching me something new about myself and the way I relate to other people. But I can't learn something from a student with whom I'm having a conflict unless I'm prepared to admit when I overreact, or when my reaction has more to do with my own psychic history than with the student's aggravating behavior.

Humbling oneself before a student requires some guts and some practice, but the rewards are significant. Students, male or female, respond to faculty respect which is genuine. A teacher's admission that she responded less than perfectly to a situation is often the opener for a student to reflect on where his own anger is coming from. Particularly in a boarding school, where she may have a student in class, in the dorm, on the athletic field and at the dinner table in one day, the teacher's job tends to cast her in the role of stand-in for the student's parent. Teachers can model emotional honesty for students—and by this I don't mean burdening students with the intimate details of one's emotional life, but simply showing that it is possible to admit when a bad day or a particular behavior drives one over the edge of patience. Dorm parents who can admit this will be more likely to hear from their students when the students' anger at faculty arises from conflicts with their parents at home, or from the bad day they just had themselves.

If good dorm parenting involves self-awareness, how does this carry over into gender issues? One thing I believe dorm parents can do is share with students their own struggle with gender issues. Male students need to hear from their male teachers and dorm parents that gender stereotyping is not just a "women's issue" but a human challenge deserving of serious attention. Students will believe that faculty really think this to the extent that they see their male teachers supporting female colleagues and encouraging female students to excel. But if male dorm parents give lip service to equal rights while denigrating girls' athletic skills or female teachers' struggles to balance career and family demands, quite a different message will be sent. Similarly, it should not be only female dorm faculty who give male boarding students the message that posters of semi-clad women in provocative poses are not appropriate decorations for the boys' dorms. Male faculty should not tolerate sexually denigrating pictures or language when they encounter them, even in the dormitory, unless they want to tell male students that respect for females need only apply in the public domain. By encouraging male students to use empathy and compassion to resolve arguments, by showing their own feelings and by respecting the vulnerabilities of students, male faculty can model behavior for male students which emphasizes interrelatedness as well as individualism.

For female faculty in female dorms, the challenges will be different. Girls need to discuss their feelings and relationships; they need straightforward information about the female reproductive cycle, its special blessings and liabilities. They also need older women to model healthy ways in which conflict can be expressed and resolved. For many adult women, anger and conflict are difficult to acknowledge; our culture still tells women it "isn't nice to be angry," and ridicules their anger when they do manage to articulate it. So adult women have a basis in their daily experience for understanding the difficulty that adolescent girls face in managing conflict. Yet women, just as much as men, are prone to use images (the "cat fight" is a classic example) which trivialize female conflicts. We need to watch out for this, to weed derogatory images out of our own conversation and call stereotyping by its rightful name wherever we encounter it, among girls or boys, students or colleagues. In particular, we need to challenge the common perception that girls' dormitories are "snake pits" of intrigue and backstabbing. They are not. But girls do use the social skills they have acquired in order to deal with problems that arise in the dorm. Observation of the nuances of human behavior and manipulation of threatening situations are the special survival skills of women in our culture. We need not denigrate girls for using these; we need to channel these skills in the direction of conflict resolution rather than continuation, camouflage and avoidance.

Faculty women who are also mothers have a special opportunity to show female students how the balance can be achieved between work and family obligations. We need to be honest about the struggle that this is, however; girls do not need to be given the impression that it must be done perfectly in order to be done at all.

Finally, if female faculty are to be perceived as serious role models, they need to exercise legitimate authority in the academic community, and they need to be supported in this task by their male colleagues. There is no surer prescription for disaster than for administrators to lace female faculty in male or female dorms without backing up their enforcement of discipline. But even if administrators do support their female faculty in this way, the message that women are secondary citizens will still be sent if there are few females in the administration itself. Because the boarding school community is such a "fish bowl" we have a unique opportunity—and challenge—to model for our students honest discussion of gender issues. Our good faith in addressing these will have more of an impact on students than any policy statements could.

Boys, Girls and Privacy

In the survey of Dublin students, girls with male dorm parents were emphatic about the issue of privacy. While they might not communicate this directly to their dorm supervisor—and, in fact, might give the impression they were less upset by inadvertent intrusions than the male faculty was—they were vehement about this concern in the anonymous questionnaire. Girls seemed to feel more exposed in a slip and stockings than boys felt in their boxer shorts in the presence of a dorm parent of the opposite sex. We socialize girls to protect themselves by covering up their bodies, so this was not a surprising finding. But it does pose a particular problem for the male dorm parent who feels the need to be a real presence in the dormitory and who wants to honor his student's right to privacy at the same time. Male faculty need to be aware of how vulnerable girls feel in less than full dress, no matter how nonchalant they act when "walked in on." Physical layout of a dormitory can exacerbate this problem and should be considered when designating dormitory use and faculty assignments. The Dublin girls who seemed most perturbed by the privacy issue lived in a dorm where some of the living space affords very little privacy if faculty are anywhere on the floor. On the other hand, a dorm parent should not allow himself to be put at a disadvantage in supervising his charges simply because they regard the entire dorm as a "bathroom-free zone." Probably the best situation is, as the female students stated, having both male and female resident faculty so that both supervision and privacy can exist side by side. Faculty spouses can also contribute enormously in this area, if they elect to be involved with the running of the dormitory.

Despite concerns about privacy, female students clearly expressed a desire for "both points of view," a "mommy figure and a daddy figure" who could provide them with feedback about the problems of daily living. Interestingly, some female students spoke about a quality of even-handedness that they appreciated in their male dorm parents and criticized some female faculty of favoritism. Perhaps the greater distance that girls felt in their relations with male dorm parents contributed to their feeling that the men were more fair. Or perhaps female students are more likely to accept male faculty as authority figures at this age when relationships between mothers and daughters can be fraught with tension. One student remarked sourly of her single female dorm parent, "She is stubborn and opinionated, and feels she must rule over us." One wonders if the same criticism would have been levelled at a male supervisor who sought to impose discipline in the dorm.

Privacy is also an issue for female faculty supervising male dormitories, although it is not perceived by male students as having such an overwhelming importance. Nevertheless, boys in the Dublin survey noted that faculty remarks to the effect of "don't worry, I've seen it all before," were dismissive of their very real embarrassment when caught on the way back from the shower clad in a towel. Again, faculty need both to knock on doors before entering, and insist that students be clothed in something more than a backward glance when they are roaming the halls between bathroom and bedroom. Female supervisors do not need to be "one of the boys" in this respect.

On the contrary, if female faculty feel comfortable taking on a "motherly" role in the dorm, that will be appreciated by their male charges. Actions speak louder than words: taking a student's temperature, brewing a pot of tea, baking a batch of cookies, all say to the individual and to the group "I care about you." It is that caring which gives any dorm parent—especially female in a male dorm—a solid basis for the use of authority. On the other hand, what's good for the gander is good for the goose: male students need to respect the limits set by the female supervisor, not only because the handbook says they must, but because they come to recognize that care must be reciprocal in order for life to be civilized.

That sense of mutual responsibility and interdependence that Gilligan says is characteristic of female moral development may be the special gift a female dorm parent has to offer her male students. Just as girls need to learn to deal with conflict more directly, boys need to develop their capacities for empathy and nurturing. A little empathy can go a long way towards reducing the amount of head-banging and hole-punching that goes on in a boys' dorm. A common project, like raising funds for something which will improve the dorm, can help to foster a greater sense of mutuality in the students living there. Allowing students to work together during study hall, instead of insisting that everyone work in splendid isolation, can do the same thing. Providing some special food for the weekly viewing of a favorite television program or dormitory meetings can weave some of the comforts of home into the daily experience of dorm life. A dormitory that feels like home is less likely to be treated like "Animal House."

The discussion of gender issues in boarding life would not be complete—or honest—unless it included some recognition of the potential for disastrous liaisons between students and faculty supervisors. Obviously, younger single faculty are more likely to be tempted to get involved in ambiguous relationships with their students, but married or older teachers are by no means exempt. Adolescents are besieged by a variety of bewildering feelings about their sexuality and social identity, just as they come into their peak years of physical energy and attractiveness. Adults who are experiencing conflict or doubt about their own social relationships may find the admiration of a particularly likeable student much simpler and more gratifying than relations with their adult equals.

When loneliness and confusion encounter unquestioning admiration, the stage is set for the not-so-mature adult to exploit the seemingly mature adolescent. What is wrong with too-intimate friendships between teachers and students, whether they become sexual relationships or not, is that the adult has stepped out of the parental role in order to enjoy an emotional closeness which belongs among equals. The teacher-student relationship is not equal as long as the student is under the teacher's authority. Too-close relationships between students and faculty breed resentment among other students and isolate the student from his peers. It is true that students often perceive younger, single faculty as more like "big brothers or sisters" than like parents. However, teachers are responsible for remembering that their function with students is parental before anything else. Schools need to provide faculty, and especially younger faculty, with very specific guidance around this issue.

Faculty also need to be aware of the nuances of gender as they enter into what are usually considered appropriate interactions with students. A male teacher may feel that he is being warmly supportive to a female student when he praises her work; but if he becomes too effusive, the student may feel it as an implied sexual overture. A female teacher who is physically demonstrative can give the wrong message by initiating hugs or patting a student on the back. But gender does not only enter into confusion over interpersonal signals. In their study of learning styles and gender, the authors of *Women's Ways of Knowing* (Belenky, Clinchy, Goldberger and Tarule, 1986) talk about how male and female pedagogical styles often differ. The "adversarial" teaching style used by many men can be intimidating to female students more at home with a collegial learning style in which synthesis, not debate, is valued. The authors also point out that, in the family, fathers are more inclined to deliver advice and fully-formed opinions to their children, while mothers are more likely to "interview" their offspring about their feelings before finalizing judgments about their behavior. Male and female dorm parents may find themselves reacting in parallel ways to their dormitory "families." Perhaps an awareness of the impact of gender on our teaching and parenting styles could offer us more choices in the ways we deal with students.

Adolescence is a time when gender identity is of paramount importance. To the extent that boarding school faculty are aware of gender issues, have wrestled with them in their personal lives, and have arrived at a comfortable sense of themselves as men and women, they will be able to help boarding students make their way through the gender-identity labyrinth. By their supportive treatment of students and colleagues, teachers act out their convictions about equality; by their capacity for nurturing and humor, they convey their acceptance of differences. My father once said to me that the older he got, the more he could see the feminine side of himself; ideally, we all come to recognize in ourselves both our gendered nature and our commonality. Living and working with adolescents requires us to examine these issues again and again. Understanding that males and females face different developmental tasks in adolescence should help us deal with our students in ways that affirm both genders.

Bibliography

Gilligan, Carol. *In a Different Voice: Psychological Theory and Women's Development.* Harvard University Press, Cambridge, MA 1982.

Belenky, Mary Field, Blythe McVicker Clinchy, Nancy Rule Goldberger and Jill Mattuck Tarule. *Women's Ways of Knowing: The Development of Self, Voice and Mind.* Basic Books, Inc., Publishers, New York, 1986.

17

The Gay/Straight Alliance

by Pamela Brown, Health Educator
Phillips Academy
Andover, Massachusetts

We call ourselves the Gay/Straight Alliance because we are all working together to make Phillips Academy as safe and as comfortable a
place to be gay, lesbian, or bisexual as it is to be heterosexual. We are
working to end homophobia as a step toward furthering the appreciation of the diversity on this campus and a stance against an oppression
which prohibits individuals from being the whole human beings that
they are.

Lofty ideals, certainly! But this description of the Phillips Academy Gay/Straight
Alliance was published in our student newspaper, *The Phillipian*, in 1990. How
did we arrive at such a place and where have we gone since? What have we
learned and what can other schools do?

It all began with a hero and an opportunity, a racial incident in the spring of
1988. The full senior class met to discuss issues of discrimination in the after-
math of the incident. Many students of color stood and shared their experiences
with racism here at school. Then a white male senior arose from the crowd and
said that it had been a tough experience for him, too, because so many students
made fun of him and didn't take him seriously because they suspected he was
gay. "Well, I am gay. If you have a problem with that, then it is your problem,
not mine." After a moment of stunned silence, the seniors began to rise; he
earned a standing ovation for his courage. Acceptance, of course, proved to be
as elusive as ever. As he went from class to class the next day not one student
mentioned the previous evening to him although they talked about it in detail
among themselves. In the end, isolation and loneliness replaced the claps and
cheers. In the name of social justice, a young man had risked everything. To
some of us in the counseling and health education departments, the challenge
was clear—we could no longer ignore the sufferings of our gay, lesbian, and
bisexual students. But what could we do?

We added a unit on homophobia to our AIDS workshops—a small step, but at least the words *gay* and *lesbian* started to be heard on campus. Then, the following year, a leader appeared in the form of an eleventh grade student who had the courage to ask her counselor to help her start a support group so that she could live honestly as the lesbian that she knew herself to be. The alternative for her was depression and despair. Without fanfare, but with great trepidation, Beth placed an announcement in the daily bulletin: "Meeting to discuss gay and lesbian rights. Tonight in the dean's meeting room. Everyone welcome."

The four adults involved in this meeting, two deans and two lesbian teachers, held our collective breaths and waited. Would anyone come? Would we get an angry response? How would the faculty react? The administration? Despite our fears and anxieties, the meeting itself was a success. Fifteen people—students, faculty, and staff—arrived and joined in a lively discussion and planning session. Beth became the president of our as yet unnamed group. The following week she penned a letter to the school newspaper; she was officially out of the closet:

> Last Tuesday evening about fifteen people met to discuss a topic that is too often ignored here at Phillips Academy. Unlike racism and sexism, nobody talks about homophobia. About ten percent of the population is homosexual and, yes, there are homosexuals at this school. It's not easy for those of us who are gay to hear our friends and classmates laugh at us or call us sick, insane, or worthy of being shot. (*The Phillipian*, February 1989)

Our club evolved as if it were a spiral. It often felt as though we were going in circles while we actually inched our way forward. A delicate balance between the needs of individual members and the needs of the group had to be found. Usually, we tipped one way and then the other. We have tried to pursue three goals simultaneously—support, education, and political action—while still managing to have fun. Striving to be inclusive rather than exclusive, we equally welcomed students and faculty, gay and straight, closet and out. Although a small, private group, we supported public events. We sought to empower individuals so that they might face the larger community with confidence and without fear. Needless to say, all of this was accomplished with minimal agreement. The only thing that we agreed on was that we should use what we had learned on the struggle against racism and sexism to fight homophobia, but the specifics always engendered a heated and lively discussion. Today, not much has changed. Our goals are the same, and we still debate every issue, but progress is visible and undeniable. Each year a few more students and faculty are comfortable being open about their sexuality.

Our membership has risen and fallen—from as high as 20 to 30 when we were the new club on the block, to as low as four or five when we became more active in challenging the status quo. In general, ten students attend our meetings. We found our name, the Gay/Straight Alliance (GSA), which expresses our desire to be open to all; we make no assumptions about our sexual orientation. This ground rule is important because we wanted to protect the privacy of those among us who are not ready to share their sexual orientation with the general public. In addition, many teenagers are not sure what their sexual orientation really is and only time and education can help them sort it out. Our students routinely place themselves in one of five categories: gay, lesbian, bisexual, straight, or confused. Straight allies are crucially important since many of our gay students face a great deal of verbal abuse from their fellows. To have straight friends who accept them openly and willingly and who support their struggles helps to heal some of this hurt. In fact, most of the time, the GSA contains more presumably straight people than gay. The primary reason here is that one's own sexuality is not an issue in the fight against homophobia. Inaction is not excused just because there are no "out" gay or lesbian faculty at a school.

There is a clear tension between our wish for openly gay and lesbian role models and our need to be non-threatening. We advertise our meetings well, but gather in an out-of-the-way place where anonymity can be assured. We don't even keep a formal membership list; only those in the club know who comes to meetings. Yet, a few of our members are very public about being lesbian or gay. These role models, both faculty and students, are extremely important for our teenagers. If one judges by movies and television, a gay person is either a psychotic killer or a transvestite. As important as it is for straight students to grow up knowing gay people, it is impossible to overstate the importance of normal gay and lesbian role models for our young homosexual students. They hunger for reassurance that they are going to have happy lives and that they are normal human beings. Nothing causes them more pain than seeing closeted faculty members who are unable to open up in the most liberal of schools. If an adult cannot be open in a liberal academic setting which espouses multiculturalism and diversity, then what hope do these youngsters have? As a result, we want more people to be "out" but, at the same time, we want to respect the privacy of those who are not ready.

The sequence of tasks that a group such as the GSA must face begins with inner work, moves to raising the consciousness of the community, and leads, ultimately, to policy changes. The faculty advisors have a number of hats to wear in this process. The inner work begins with private counseling and support for individuals while education is provided for everyone within the group. Speakers are found for some of our meetings. The most successful topics have been coming out stories by alumni, alcoholism by gay members of Alcoholics Anonymous, and issues for gay people of color. Someone must research information on gay literature and history, find out about good movies, and learn of events that the group can celebrate. This leads naturally to the second function: raising community awareness. We now have an annual Gay Awareness Week that culminates with National Coming Out Day. We all have pink triangle stickers to give out along with a short lesson about the history of gay rights. Pink triangles were worn by gay prisoners awaiting execution in German concentration camps in World War II. Today, gay rights and AIDS activists have adopted the symbol. We place a pink triangle in every tenth mail box on campus, and we explain that approximately ten percent of our population is either gay, lesbian, or bisexual. We put together biographies of magazine articles. We provide these packets of information to anyone who wants to learn more about gay issues. However, the most successful events are the conferences and social events that bring students from many schools together. Our annual conference here at Phillips Academy brings together 75 students and faculty from a dozen or so New England private and public schools. Many students or teachers come from schools in which they are the only person who is dealing with issues of homosexuality. After spending a weekend with so many others committed to the same cause, one is simultaneously reluctant to leave yet anxious to return home to spread the news. Emotions are strong, spirits are renewed, and hope is rekindled.

At our student's urging, the school has included sexual orientation in its statement of non-discrimination that is printed in the school catalogue and faculty and staff handbooks. We have brought up the issues of spousal equivalency so that gay and lesbian faculty members may live in campus housing with their partners. This proposed policy change has been presented to the board of trustees so the whole cycle of education, awareness, consciousness raising, and policy change is happening there as well. We have a dream of someday having gay individuals and couples running dorms and living as freely and openly as do our heterosexual colleagues.

At this point, I always have to crash back to the real world. The vision is so clear that I can almost kid myself into thinking that it is reality. Every step that we take feels like such a victory and such a gain that hope and enthusiasm overtakes common sense. The ultimate irony is that the reticence of our gay and lesbian faculty members to help in this effort is the strongest indicator of how much remains to be done. Until gays and lesbians feel fully accepted by society, they will hide. After all, this is not an issue of hiring gay and lesbian faculty members; they are already here! Instead, the issue is creating a safe environment in which they can be open. The problem is in the straight world and its response to homosexuality. Inevitably, the solution will have to come from the heterosexual world too. Straight people must speak out in concert with gays, lesbians, and bisexuals to demand an educational system that educates for justice, harmony, and social change. Then, and only then, will our students grow up with positive self-images, free of the damaging isolation and fear that defines and confines their lives today.

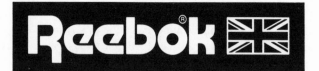

TENNIS CAMPS

Under the direction of Dartmouth Men's Tenn
Coach Chuck Kinyon, the Reebok Tennis Camps off
a wide range of tennis camping experiences.

For the younger set (ages 10 - 17), the Reebo
Junior Tennis Camp weeks offer 5 - 6 hours of dai
instruction and supervised play, team tenn
competition, video tape analysis of each playe
games, with several innovative teaching techniqu
enabling every participant the opportunity
improve and develop their tennis game towa
reaching their ultimate potential.

For the more mature crowd, the Reebok Adu
Tennis Camp weeks use the same instructional ba
as the very successful Junior Weeks, but with a
more emphasis on playing strategies.

If you would like a detailed brochure regarding t
Reebok Tennis Camps, please write:

Reebok Tennis Camps
c/o Chuck Kinyon, DCAD
6083 Alumni Gymnasium
Hanover, NH   03755-3512

or call: (603) 646-3819

THE
pump
TM

18

Faculty of Color

by Michael Williamson, Director of Student Activities
Germantown Friends School
Philadelphia, Pennsylvania

Reflections On My Own Experience

Life for a young adult living at a boarding school can be heaven or hell. For a person of color the additional burden of race and living in a predominantly white environment is an added complication. My experience indicates that there is good will and good intention in the independent school world for making diversity a top priority. However, the fact that the independent school world remains overwhelmingly white, wealthy and privileged with a culture focused on academic, social and economic exclusivity and legacy is inescapable. By design, it is not for everyone.

My wife and I were married in June of 1981 at the Fox School Meetinghouse and set up a household in the boys dorm called Pennswood that same summer. My wife lived in a girl's dorm at Fox the year preceding our marriage and as dean was required to live on campus. Therefore our living arrangement from the outset was a matter of convenience for the school. My wife, an alumna of a progressive New England boarding school, spoke of these four best years of her life often; her enthusiasm countered my reservations. Before marriage I was living in a house I renovated in Philadelphia in an urban, struggling, predominantly black community where I, in fact, had little in common with my aging, working class neighbors. I worked in a small, K-6 independent alternative school. As a native of Philadelphia, I attended public school for 13 years until college. The only people I knew who went to boarding schools were those whose parents were in the process of splitting up or kids who "got into trouble." The options were intriguing. Living in the country, in a dormitory and working with young people was appealing to me. In addition I was starting a new teaching job at a K-12 girl's school on the Main Line so I knew I would encounter the "outside world" daily.

In September 1981 I began teaching at Regal School by day and supervising ten boys in the Pennswood Dorm of 70 boys in the evenings and every fifth weekend. The head of Pennswood was a 12-year veteran of the dorm when we moved in. There were three other hall teachers. One, like me, was not teaching at the school and was new to the boarding school experience. The other two had been at the school for two or three years. Each of the four halls had a pair of prefects who helped maintain order during the evening study hall and helped with check-in. The dorm head, the hall teachers and prefects met once a week to share specific concerns about study hall conditions, social and disciplinary issues, clean- up procedures, and ideas for special ''all-dorm'' activities such as pizza parties and intra-dorm team sport contests.

As younger faculty with no children, much of the school year was consumed by our involvement in teaching, preparing for classes, monitoring study halls, transporting and getting to know students and providing a surrogate home when the need arose. Given the location of our apartment and our own temperaments we were seen by the boys as almost always available. Most evenings during study hall and at check-in our dining room door would be open. Some evenings at check-in we made popcorn and it became a ritual for the boys to get to us as early as possible for a snack and conversation.

During the first few months of living in the dorm my wife and I worked at adjusting to married life, my commute, a new job and getting acquainted with the students and faculty in the dorm. I have been told that the most stressful activities in early adulthood are getting married, moving, and starting a new job. Within these short months I had done all three . . . and lived with 70 teenage boys.

Working With Faculty

Other than getting to know 70 boys by first name during the first three weeks of school, the most difficult adjustment was learning to co-exist with the other adults in the dorm.

Soon after settling into our apartment, Hal, the dorm head, invited my wife and I to his family's apartment for dinner. It was clear that we were all embarking on a new relationship which would be intimate, complex, necessarily cordial and not without its peculiar stresses. During the first few weeks our families spent time together—bowling, playing tennis, going out for pizza, doing laundry (we all shared the student laundry area), having dinner in the dining room and attending various school functions. The relationship with the boss was more intimate by necessity than what most work situations require. I knew from the outset that we shared much less in common naturally and that it was truly fate and only fate that brought us together. On the surface we interacted as equals although it was clear who ran the show in the dorm. The intimacy of boarding school life can be overwhelming. It was not long before we had too intimate a knowledge of one another's nervous tics, idiosyncracies and shortcomings. The depth of our commitment to kids and to the necessity of supporting one another through difficult dorm issues would unfold over the course of this first year.

The intimacy of dorm life, knowing and being known by all, demands hours of commitment. It is not uncommon to be awakened at two in the morning from a deep sleep because a student is ill, lonely, there is a fire drill, or the students have staged an impromptu raid to greet the first snowfall of the season. The routine of the dorm determines the rhythm of your personal life. Often it shapes you more than you shape it. If I had been single, this would have been an unthinkable prospect.

For a young, single person, especially a black person in a predominantly white environment, the dating and social scene is tentative at best. Implicit is an understanding that single faculty be discreet, modest, and a role model for the young at all times. An overnight guest was permissible but "no steamer trunks." Any faculty member with an overnight guest was the topic of conversation at the faculty breakfast table the following morning. It was a given that the students knew the sleeping, drinking, smoking and sexual habits of the dorm faculty. Students know more about faculty habits than the converse.

Trust

As a monogamous, married black man my intimate life was probably less suspect and less interesting to students and faculty than if I had been single. Still as the only adult black couple on campus we were a minor curiosity to students and our colleagues. I felt my actions were scrutinized and more closely monitored by the dorm head, especially in the beginning, than my white colleagues. I have heard this comment from other blacks working in independent schools. It is a disturbing perception but not a wholly surprising one. It is more likely that a black person working at an independent school has lived or interacted with whites prior to their independent school experience. In the case of my dorm head, it was the first time he had a black neighbor. The intimacy of boarding school life demands a basic level of trust and communication among the dorm faculty. There is, on a larger societal level, little trust between blacks and whites and there is no reason to assume the independent school world is an exception.

I can only speculate about Hal's apprehensions but I know I bristled at the level of control dorm life imposed on me. For example the dorm head has a master key to all faculty apartments. Late one afternoon as my wife was finishing her shower in preparation for an outing with Hal and his family, there was a buzz at the entrance door. Scantily attired, not yet ready to receive a visitor, my wife was astounded to meet Hal partway between the front door and our dining room. I suspected that he had used his master key. I was deeply troubled by this and let him know it directly. He said the door was ajar and thought it was alright to come in. I made it clear that he was not to enter our apartment without prior permission and that his power as a dorm head did not extend beyond our threshold. What "good-natured" Hal saw as neighborly intimacy we saw as an appalling invasion of privacy. It was unfortunate that Hal walked into our apartment without our formal greeting and it was unfortunate that I assumed his means of entry and motive were untoward. Clearly we had both made an assumption that violated the sense of trust, privacy, and familial intimacy that is part of the unwritten culture of the boarding school.

Support and Evaluation

The hidden culture of the independent school can lead to misunderstandings about community expectations of faculty. For faculty of color unfamiliar with residential school life, the multifaceted role as teacher, coach, mentor to students, professional colleague within an academic department and establishing adult friendships may seem overwhelming and unclear. Nuts and bolts information can be found in the faculty handbook about policy, procedures and responsibility but wisdom concerning budgeting time, setting limits for student behavior in the classroom, dorm or playing field, forming meaningful but appropriate and healthy relationships with students can best be gleaned from supportive, experienced faculty. How much time with students is too much? What is the average number of hours a new teacher spends each evening preparing for the following day's classes? After a full day of classes, coaching, dinner in the dining room, monitoring an evening study hall how do you muster the energy or motivation to grade papers or write reports? These are the issues that affect all younger faculty struggling with balance and order in settling into school life. These pressures will be more acute for those isolated faculty of color.

Establishing a tone in the classroom, the dorm, or the playing field can be a natural or acquired skill but undoubtedly an essential one for effective teaching and learning. Will the children of privilege who inhabit our schools instantly accord a young woman or man of color the same level of respect accorded a white teacher? Are you sure? When and how is it appropriate to lose one's temper with students? How, within the culture of your school, is anger, frustration and dismay expressed?

I have found that younger faculty of color who are intimate with the students of color run the risk of being perceived as too close to students by their white colleagues. On closer examination it becomes clear that the bond between younger faculty of color and students of color is strong because the chasm of experience between black and white adults is often so deep and broad. Students are more welcoming and inclusive.

Boarding schools with a deliberate process of support and evaluation for all new teachers, that is mindful of the additional pressures on faculty of color working in a predominantly white institution, are poised to preempt teacher fatigue. The system that is timely and ongoing, which includes a buddy system, one or two faculty members who have the time and inclination to take one new faculty member under their wing, should include professional and social support. The most useful evaluation process is one that affirms the good work of the faculty and provides clear and useful pedagogy. An atmosphere in which the teacher and the supervisor can share successes and frustrations freely, clearly, directly, helpfully and fairly is what we all want and deserve.

Assumptions

I remember a conversation with a dorm teacher, after several sets of Ping-Pong, that extended into the wee hours of the morning. The subject evolved into a frank discussion of race and racism. Most striking to me was that this white, friendly, intelligent, prep school-educated denizen of Greenwich, Connecticut and Dartmouth graduate struggled to convince me that racism did not exist anymore, except in some remote, backwoods areas. I could not convince him, partly because of his unswerving arrogance, that just because I come from a family whose sons were educated at Yale, that I cannot stand apart from the masses of black people who are yet to be accorded equity and justice in this society. Because he and I had so much in common with a privileged lifestyle he assumed his experience of the world was also mine. There is an element of the boarding school experience where class distinction and material inequities disappear for faculty and students. However egalitarian the living arrangements appear, the leveling effect of the boarding experience does not transcend the pervasive societal discomfort with frank conversation about issues of race.

Member of the Club

There are issues that sometimes affect the people of color at a boarding school that go unnoticed by the white faculty and students. For the assembly program to honor the birth of Dr. Martin Luther King, I was asked to make some introductory remarks. I read an excerpt from the "I Have A Dream" speech and posed several questions to the audience to contemplate how we had yet to live out this dream. Among the eight questions was "Why can't I get a haircut in Middletown?" There was an audible "oh yeah" from the boys and girls of color in the audience. I did not see this as a particularly provocative question or one that in answering was cause for debate. I knew from my own experience and from the experience of current boys in our dorm that either you went to another town to get a haircut or one of the other black students cut your hair. I had bought a set of clippers and these were circulated throughout the dorm. I had a standing appointment with an enterprising young black man from my dorm who cut my hair. Had I ever gone to the white barbers in Middletown? No. Did any of my white colleagues who frequented "Phil's" or "Dave's" see any black patrons in the shop? Did any white faculty ask black kids where they received their haircuts? I was challenged by several angry faculty and the head of school because they felt my remark was unsubstantiated. "Of course Phil cuts black peoples' hair!" "If you've never been to Phil's how do you know he wouldn't cut your hair?" Only one faculty member who spoke with me, a resident of the town for more than 20 years, said I was absolutely right. She added that in the late 70s Phil had refused to cut a black student's hair and a group of black students responded by mounting a peaceful picket in front of the shop. Why didn't any of the senior faculty remember this? Why was I immediately accused of lying? Does one need to test the waters and be insulted to prove discrimination? Why was the black experience immediately suspect? Are there faculty or administrators at the school who stand to validate the experiences of students of color?

Tradition

One of a series of events on the annual Parents' Day was the afternoon tea at the headmaster's house. This was attended by most parents and was designed so that they could get to know one another and talk with the head of school and the faculty in an informal setting. I was asked by the head after one of these events why there were so few black parents in attendance. He felt the informality of the event and his own straightforward manner generally made people comfortable. I agreed. However I had to point out that for a number of families of color his palatial home and patrician ease might be intimidating. Many of these parents in their mid-40s or 50s had no prior experience with the prep school world, unless they had worked on the grounds crew or in the kitchen. The orientation for parents, the teacher conferences and the luncheon may be far less intimidating than the social and more intimate tea. How often do adults of different racial, religious and economic classes interact on a social level? What might the conversation be like between the black auto mechanic and the white president of Yale?

Alumni day at schools can be an event that is both inviting and exclusionary. Until the last 20 years or so, few independent schools had substantial numbers of students of color. To view rows and rows of alumni photographs without a trace of anyone who looks like you underscores the covert issues of race in the history of our schools. The visual reminder of exclusion is in odd contrast to the joyful reverie of the white alumni who speak fondly of the past. It is useful for current students of color and faculty of color to interact with recent alumni, especially alumni of color, as their experiences, positive and negative, help foster a continuum that is so much a part of the independent school experience. New traditions need to be included that reflect the changing constituencies within the school.

Diversity within Diversity

During the eight years I spent living in the dorm and working in a boarding school it was a challenge to look at each student as an individual with his or her own unique personality and set of experiences and not typecast them or prejudge what appeared to be a predictable scenario. Looking back at the students of color I have known, I realize much of their personal history, family background and experience of Fox School was not widely solicited, known, understood or valued by the faculty. This is not to imply that the individual was not valued but the idea that the diverse experiences students bring with them is a valuable offering to the larger school community is mostly an afterthought—a by-product of the quest to "better" the lives of the disadvantaged. It was often the case that the black students' experience of school, the gap they had to bridge between the world of home and the world of school, was mostly unknown to the adults at the school. For many students, regardless of color, the boarding experience allows them to be seen as a *tabula rasa*. Again it is assumed by the members of the residential school that students and faculty of color share this privileged, rarified academic and culturally rich environment and our experience of it is similar, good and of exquisite value; my experience is your experience.

A look at the profiles of several students of color reveals diversity within diversity which goes beyond skin color. Beyond this veneer is the more subtle but no less tangible consideration of class and ethnicity among people of color.

A closer look at black boys at Fox School reveals a wide range of experiences predicated on class and ethnicity as an important subset of race. The range of backgrounds of the students of color during my years at Fox School was as rich and varied as that of the white students: "celebrity brat," "international diplomat kid," "international bi-racial," "American bi-racial," "urban street kid," "middle class, suburban, two parents," "immigrant," "first generation American," "raised by a grandparent," "athlete-scholar," "single parent household," "academic star," "popular All-American." Unfortunately and too often I heard comments from faculty that began with or included "Well the black kids are . . ." or "these kids are really different . . ." or "I can't relate to these kids . . ." The "I can't relate" is especially aggravating to me. If schools responded to this with, "Relate or seek employment elsewhere," I am sure white faculty would, with their insight, resources and intelligence, initiate the kind of dialogue and conversation that would begin to bridge the gap between our diverse experiences. It is our business to facilitate learning by disseminating information in ways that engage kids, all kids. As a black faculty member it is a given that I am expected to relate to white kids and exist as a role model with special insights into the world of kids of color. Shouldn't all faculty work to the best of their ability for all students?

Ask, Don't Assume

It is important to realize that much of the negative baggage kids of color carry with them is not easily shared with adults. If the immediate reaction is, "It can't happen here," then why tell the story. It is very difficult to share a humiliating experience when the audience is doubting or too quick to trivialize the experience. A number of white faculty at our school were amazed at the range of stories black and white kids shared when we undertook the Multicultural Assessment Plan devised by NAIS. There were a number of instances of black and white kids together in Middletown shopping or getting pizza who were verbally assaulted with racial epithets hailed from drivers along the highway. On numerous occasions black kids were followed in the shops by overzealous clerks who assumed our kids would shoplift. Sometimes wholly unsubstantiated accusations were made or black kids were just told to "get out." These were often the very same shops that so graciously served our faculty. Our school quickly realized that no one was asking the question of students, "What is your experience of the racial climate at this school and the surrounding environs?"

In Loco Parentis

Often kids of color were invited to the homes of white students for the weekend and felt the sting of parental surprise and disdain at their child's choice of a weekend guest. There were also instances of gracious white families inviting kids of color to their country club, a club that would tolerate them as a guest but not as a member. This kind of subtle humiliation is difficult for any adolescent to wrestle with alone. Adults need to be there for them to talk with, to share their anger and to stand together against the bastions of intolerance and humiliation. It is very important for adults from the school to be clear in stating that discrimination is wrong. It is imperative that kids, both black and white, know exactly where the school stands as they can easily see ambivalence as compromise. Students of color should not be compromised. White guilt and black victimhood do not help but only stand in the way of identifying, confronting and changing attitudes and bigotry.

Our Blood Is Red

Dating is a major issue with the kids of color living at a boarding school. Most of the black boys I knew at Fox School curiously did not have steady girlfriends though they were popular. There were some inter-racial couples, black boys with white girls mostly. There were some strong taboos against inter-racial dating that many black kids brought from home and this was reinforced by their black peers. Inter-racial dating in the black community has often been associated with a repudiation of one's skin color and cultural heritage. Some black girls would be most vociferous about their anger at some black guys for dating white girls. This struck at the very core of the black girls' evolving self-esteem as the archetype of feminine beauty in our culture is fair haired and blue eyed. Some didn't care. There were a small handful of white boys that dated black girls. I never heard any white girls make remarks about this. I think the dating scene for black girls at the school was often quite grim as they were competing with white girls and black girls for the sparse black males.

The multicultural student organization would sponsor a dance once a year that was attended by most kids on campus. It was a very real celebration of black popular culture at school and the dancing and the music was pulsating and lively.

It was an accepted fact that at this once-a-year activity everyone danced and it was fun.

Independent schools are bound by mission statements. A common thread in these statements is our striving to educate young people to think and to act in accord with specific moral and ethical codes. Schools are where young people from a wide range of social, economic, ethnic and racial backgrounds can learn about one another and come to respect, honor and value difference. The boarding school *in loco parentis* has the added responsibility of around-the-clock commitment. Residential schools must engineer the social context of the boarding experience to match the quality academic program which prepares young people to act in the world for positive change.

Recommendations

- Boarding schools need faculty of color to help students of all colors to bridge the gap of their limited experiences in segregated America.
- Boarding schools need faculty of color to help dispel assumptions the privileged have about "the masses" and "the real world."
- Boarding schools need to reflect in their dorm staff, faculty, administration and governing board the diversity of experience that is already becoming an element of the student body.
- The orientation to boarding schools for students and parents should include workshops, exercises or small discussion groups that focus on the adjustment to boarding life. Class and racial differences should be addressed directly.
- We need to attend to the social life of the kids of color at boarding schools. Their needs are different because their options are fewer. Most adolescents long for the perceived "true" high school experience: romance and dances. The fond memories students have of their boarding school experience is predicated on the richness and depth of the friendships made.
- Networking among other boarding and day schools in the area with their students of color broadens the social pool for students of color. Students of color may love square dancing, apple picking, folk music and golf but also seek their ideas on selecting and arranging special activities that reflect their interests and culture.
- Anticipate anger and confusion from students of color over issues of discrimination. Expect students in moments of crisis to respond with a full range of emotions encompassing rational and irrational behavior. Listen. Accept the fact that you may not be an expert on race relations. It's OK.
- Undertake the Multicultural Assessment Plan adopted by NAIS. It is a useful instrument for getting students, faculty, administration and board leadership thinking about the practices of the school as well as the academic

program and school climate as it concerns people of color and the white majority.

- A system of support and evaluation for new faculty should include professional development and formal and informal liaisons to the faculty social network. The faculty social network is crucial to orienting faculty of color new to independent schools.

19

Toward a Multicultural School

by Jan Gilley, Dean of Students &
International Student Advisor
Westover School
Middlebury, Connecticut

On a warm day in late August the blue van pulled up to our school entrance where several faculty members and their children were waiting. Inside the van sat two smiling but tired looking girls surrounded by large suitcases and heavily taped boxes covered with Chinese or Japanese characters. Not being familiar with these languages, I found myself guessing, trying to decide which girls had arrived, the two from Shanghai or the two from Tokyo. Our new homestay program was about to begin.

The girls tumbled off the van, and amid warm but timid welcomes the new-comers said their names, making it obvious that our Chinese girls had arrived. They looked a little bewildered and definitely shy. We took most of their be-longings to the dormitory rooms, while they held on to a suitcase for the home-stay. Within 24 hours all 15 new international students had arrived and had been packed off to the homes of faculty or day students to rest and to begin exploring their new temporary homeland. From cities with millions of people, they had come to live in a world of 155 girls and about 50 adults. From tiny apartments in Tokyo, tidy homes in Sweden, and sunny cities in Africa they came to live with us in rural New England.

Our school had decided in the spring that new international students needed a buffer between their homes and our school. Other schools offer similar programs to their students, but we had decided that a small home situation would be the most gentle way to begin to absorb a new culture. The three-day stay was just long enough for the young bodies to overcome jet lag, to adjust to the strange water, and to sample a few new foods. It was also long enough to get acquainted with at least one adult who would be a constant in this curious place, and to begin the exchange of customs and cultures which would, we hoped, be a life-changing experience for all concerned.

Although most boarding schools have histories of educating students from other countries, until recent years the numbers of these students were very small and were limited to children of American parents living abroad or children of the wealthy and powerful. As we are diversifying our American student bodies, so the make-up of our international groups is also cutting across more social and economic classes. We now serve children of secretaries from Shanghai, engineers from Germany, and travel agents from Spain as well as the children of royal households. What an amazing opportunity! On our small campuses we have more diversity than in most larger schools in major urban areas. Most of us have American students from inner city areas, suburbia and rural areas who come from an array of economic, religious and racial backgrounds. When added to our American students, the international students become one more resource for learning that can be a great advantage to our communities.

The diversity that we should esteem is not always looked upon favorably by students or faculty. There are problems inherent in any institution that attempts to make a unified community in the face of so much diversity. In these problems we find our challenges and our opportunities. The treatment of our students, both American and international, should have careful consideration. The assimilation of our international students into an already heterogeneous group takes sensitive and careful planning.

Several years ago, during a flight to Hong Kong, I tried to pinpoint the interest I have always had in people of different races and cultures other than my own. A picture flashed into my mind. It was one which had hung in my room when I was very young, and depicted a group of children. I remembered studying the faces of those children who were black and Asian and Indian and Native American and Eskimo, and wondering where there were such faces—certainly not in my town. Later in life, as I studied geography and read *National Geographic* from cover to cover, my interest continued. All this time I marveled at the wonders of one culture after another discovered on the pages of this unique magazine. I longed to visit them and to know someone whose life was so different from mine.

This early admiration for the marvelous diversity of our earth has helped to form my belief that one goal of a multicultural school must be just that: to be multicultural. For most boarding schools the evolution to levels of great diversity was completely unplanned. It has just happened that we have the variety of human resources that we do. We must remember that having diversity does not automatically mean that we have a multicultural school. We must work toward that end. Our task would be much easier if we, who take students from many countries, could simply attempt to Americanize them. To shed the garb of the old culture and robe in the style of the new would be a great deal less complicated than the task at hand. But, I am confident that Americanizing our international students should not be our goal. There is far more to be gained by the entire school community when the goal of international education is to help all students feel comfortable in and understand more than one culture. It is essential that we build not just tolerance for other beliefs and customs, but interest in them and respect for them. The Americanization of international students may be a goal of schools who are working with immigrants to this country, but, even so, it should not be the only goal, for the narrowness of this goal is not in the best interests of the students or the school.

Assuming that the goal of international education on the secondary level is for a student to become multi- or bicultural, how then is the educational and boarding process organized to this end? The academic learning at our school is done entirely in English (except in foreign language classes). A great deal of the literature we study is of the Western world. The academic life of the school can be enriched by the addition of international students as well as burdened by their needs. Most schools who take these students have an English as a Second Language program in place, but sometimes only the Americanization of the international students is served by ESL. Finding comfortable ways to share the cultures of our visiting students is also a goal we should approach seriously. Preparing international students to speak, read and write English well enough to satisfy the requirements of our regular curriculum and earn a diploma is certainly one goal of English as a Second Language, and a constant concern of our academic offices. A second goal of no less importance should be to help international students find comfort in our culture and recognize that they have something to offer us as we have something to offer them. The fact that we work with secondary school students means that we have more opportunity to set the stage for excellent multicultural exchange.

The ESL teacher must be a person who truly believes in multicultural education and should be carefully selected for her sensitivity to the difficulties of adjustment. She needs to be able to establish the kind of comfort level in the classroom which allows students to feel free enough to ask the questions they need to ask. One of the most trying situations for a young person who does not speak English very well is that of hearing others around her laughing and not knowing what the laughter is about. Both American and international students who have good English skills are not always thoughtful of the struggling international students and don't take time to explain situations. Certainly in the beginning, the ESL teacher needs to serve as one who helps students understand what is happening on a daily basis.

There are many ways in which the ESL teacher can ease the adjustment to our country and particularly to the school. Although my purpose is not to write a "how to" manual, a few suggestions should illustrate helpful activities. The ESL teacher should explain upcoming holidays, school events, and general customs. These explanations can be worked into the curriculum and serve as exercises in language skills. Assigned interviews with American students and faculty members can be on topics such as "How Americans Celebrate Thanksgiving," or "What is the Most Important School Tradition?" or "Why Do Some Teachers Prefer Being Called By Their First Names." By working in the interview process the international student is forced into the community to seek answers to questions which must be asked of Americans. This forced interaction can be a very valuable experience. The ESL teacher can keep ahead of things which are happening in the school and make certain that the international students feel comfortable taking part in school life by giving them some prior understanding of the activities. The explanations given to all students by student leaders and others are usually not enough. Often explanations given in large assembly or lecture halls do not reach the international student at all. They are frequently not loud or clear enough.

One Halloween I had two nervous Chinese students approach me to ask what a "costume parade" was. They had heard the announcement by student leaders in assembly, but had no idea what was going to happen. I explained the Halloween tradition and tried to give them some ideas about dressing up in costume. When I realized that they were still very unsure about all of this and were looking very discouraged, I tried to think of storybook characters they might have read about in their early study of English. They said that they had read some children's stories. When I mentioned "Little Red Riding Hood," they beamed and nodded their heads. I suggested that they dress up like two of the characters in the story. The sad expressions returned to their faces. Obviously, they really didn't have the things they would need to make costumes. Off we ran to my attic and found enough old clothing to create Red Riding Hood and the grandmother. They asked if I would lend them my dog to play the wolf and then hastily returned to the school to join the parade, giggling as they ran.

Another way that international students can be made to feel comfortable, both with their native culture and with their new culture, is to keep bulletin boards or notebooks with articles about things of importance which are happening in their countries. The educational benefits of looking through newspapers and magazines and then explaining to classmates the importance of the events reported there are great. This research and reading assignment, while in English, can help international students stay connected with their homelands.

One of the most meaningful moments in my teaching experience happened during the reunification of Germany. The four German students at our school were following the television and newspaper news during every free minute. Two West Germans girls had been very involved with a church project which sent necessities to groups in East Germany. One student had relatives in East Germany whom she had never met. They asked if they could put on a short assembly for the school about how they were feeling. Since several of the girls were dancers, a ballet was created to tell their story. The school was treated to a lovely and moving performance, which not only gave the German girls a chance to express their delight and their fears, but gave the Americans a chance to gain a real understanding of this historic event. The emotional impact on the community was very powerful.

Just as a school would not consider offering to teach ballet when they do not have a ballet teacher or AP calculus when they do not have a qualified mathematics teacher, neither should it offer to take international students, in any numbers, unless they have a program in place for these students. Most schools can handle several exchange students in a given year, but groups of international students need attention and special teaching, especially in the beginning. An international student advisor should plan to spend a great deal of time with the group and with individuals during the adjustment time. It is my experience that weekly meetings, which are necessary at first, taper off to monthly meetings toward the beginning of the second half of the year. European, Mexican and South American students seem to need active support for a shorter period of time than Asian students. As the language usually takes the Asian students longer to master, so total adjustment seems more difficult.

Although international students need to be convinced about the validity of learning English if they are to survive in our schools, they must not be made to feel that their native language and culture is unimportant. We must never neglect the opportunity to pull cultures together and to encourage mutual respect and understanding. There are many projects and assignments which creative teachers can initiate if they remember that another goal of the program is to educate students who function well in more than one culture and who have respect for all people. Many schools hold international dinners or encourage students to speak about life in their countries. These activities are good experiences for both the international students who have to use English in their explanations and Americans who learn about another way of life. The same opportunity can be given to American students from different regions of our country to share any of their culture.

The work of a talented ESL teacher can certainly make a big difference in the adjustment of new international students to a school, but the rest of the faculty has to be involved in the process also. Departments must agree about the expectations of these students. Teachers, advisors, academic deans and deans of students need to be able to work as a team with the international student advisor to solve problems which arise with these students. The complications, for example, of discussing academic or social problems with visiting parents who do not speak English may require the hiring of an interpreter. Because it is sometimes difficult to assess the level of English ability or other academic abilities, we occasionally find students in our classes who are poorly equipped to handle our workload. When it is ascertained that an international student will not be able to meet the expectations of our schools, the difficulties encountered in helping the family find an alternative educational plan for the child demand great teamwork. Since parents may be halfway around the world, this can be a very complicated venture. The fax machine has been a great help to many schools in dealing with international students and parents. A school should also seek out professional resources among local people who are bi- or multi-lingual. I have had the good fortune to find such people in several of the urban areas near our school. These people are often willing to talk to parents, explain problems which we are incapable of communicating because of language or cultural barriers, and find solutions.

The problems of disciplinary situations with American children whose parents speak English are often difficult enough. In situations with international students who have gotten into serious trouble, the problems multiply. The inability to communicate directly with parents who will be embarrassed and humiliated by their child's behavior requires some understanding of "face-saving" tactics. If these parents are unfamiliar with the American education system, they may not understand our disciplinary system at all. In addition if they are unfamiliar with the use of social workers and psychologists in helping students who are reacting to extremely stressful situations, they will not understand the use of counseling or therapy.

Early one school year, a student who was doing good academic work, was caught with items which had been taken from other students and teachers. She would not admit to having stolen the items and seemed to be confused as to how they got into her room. She went through the normal disciplinary process but was accused of lying to the disciplinary committee. There was a question in my mind about whether or not she understood the procedure or the questions asked of her.

In this case we needed the help of some outside professionals who evaluated the student and told us that they believed she was experiencing a kind of culture shock. Not only did they help evaluate the child, they admitted her to their program for some time and tried to give her skills to deal with her emotional needs. She did very well in that therapeutic community with the help of the doctors and the faculty members from our school who visited her. In the psychiatrists' opinion, she was indeed experiencing a kind of culture shock, but they also said that the problem could be much more complicated. We brought her back to school after a few weeks, but in the end found that we could not manage her. Because our school does not keep students after a repeated major offense and because we are not an institution equipped to handle major emotional problems, we had to make arrangements to send this student home. This process was more difficult than I had anticipated. The parents were unwilling to have her sent home. We finally agreed to send her to some relatives in another state and through follow-up phone calls learned that she eventually was sent home. During this time we learned the importance of the support system which we established for the international students. That support system includes the dean, our social worker, an outside consultant psychiatrist, translators and, of course, the dormitory parents.

Helpful people outside the school community are sometimes difficult to find.

When I needed help, I began by calling all of the people I knew who might be able to steer me to the person I needed. The local hospital helped me find a psychiatrist who spoke the language I needed; an experienced admission person helped me find a psychiatric hospital; a clergyman helped me find a local couple who could provide support for a homesick child. Our parents' committee and our alumnae groups helped to find homestays and summer jobs. Sometimes it seemed as if I spent days on the phone, but the support for the needs of these students was found both on and off campus.

The dormitory parents are the most important contacts for the international students outside the classroom. Their daily care and interventions in times of need are essential to a good program. Special training for both classroom and dormitory faculty can help sensitize them to the needs and problems of international students. We have used a film produced by Boston University called *Cold Water* to educate our staff about the feelings of students coming from other cultures and to generate discussions which lead to a deeper understanding of our students. Our school social worker and dean of faculty helped organize and run the discussions with both faculty and student leaders. There are workshops offered every year across our country which can be helpful to people who work with international students.

Most schools receive mailings from some of the groups which sponsor these workshops. At national and regional meetings of independent schools there are usually sessions which have to do with international students. NAFSA: Association of International Educators, which has been involved mainly on the college level, is beginning to have an active group of secondary school educators. Although their newsletter is often focused on issues which affect higher education and older students, there are articles of interest to all who are concerned with multicultural education. They also carry in their newsletter advertisements for health insurance for international students and books and pamphlets for the use of faculty. Their address is: 1875 Connecticut Avenue, N.W. Suite 1000, Washington, D.C. 20009-5728. Places like the Intercultural Press in Yarmouth, Maine, also offer many books helpful to educators, parents and students.

Any available school year workshops or summer sessions could be invaluable in the training of dormitory parents. The dormitory parents, in particular, need training and support to help them deal with their own communication frustrations and those of their young charges. It can be very helpful to choose a book about working with international students on the secondary level and use it as a basis for discussion at several dorm parent meetings. Problems, large and small, can be avoided with the right training and information. Dorm parents can benefit greatly by recognizing small problems which can cause larger problems. Simple things like learning to use coin-operated washing machines and getting over a fear of the health center are only two of the many situations which can be very difficult in the early weeks for international students. A student who avoids doing laundry can get into trouble with a roommate or classmates for causing unpleasant odors in bedrooms and classrooms. A student who avoids the health center can get very sick if a respiratory infection or other disease goes untreated.

It is normal for the international students to go through stages of adjustment to this culture, and awareness of the stages can help the faculty understand the changes these students are experiencing. The excitement of the early days gives way to homesickness and sometimes later even depression and anger. It takes an enormous amount of mental and emotional energy to live in a foreign environment and communicate in a foreign language 24 hours a day. There is a point when all of the struggle of keeping up in another language becomes overwhelming, and the student is exhausted and sometimes even begins to hate everything American. One of the most difficult times of the year for these students is after Christmas vacation, especially those who come from warm climates. I am not sure that we New Englanders realize the challenge that winters are for those who are not used to them. I took a group of students on a cross country train trip during one spring break. We began by visiting Washington, D.C. and ended in Colorado for some skiing. During a particularly long day, as we were walking from the Smithsonian toward the Lincoln Memorial, I was teasing the group about how slowly they were walking on their young legs. They protested greatly and said that the walking didn't bother them, but they had quite enough of the cold and the wind. We compromised on a taxi ride back to the hotel! By the time we got to the skiing, the late March sun in Colorado was a real pleasure for them.

Aside from the social and language adjustments, the international student also has to adjust to the American methods of teaching and learning. Asking questions and speaking out in our small classes are new skills for most of them. Writing lengthy papers is a trip through uncharted waters. Competitive academics are a new experience to students for whom cooperative methods have been the norm. The American concern over plagiarism is a concept that is extremely difficult for international students to understand. As a colleague and I conversed about a case of possible plagiarism, she offered the following explanation of why the idea of plagiarism might be so difficult, especially for Asian students:

> When my child's third grade teacher asks her to make a chart about the weather in the rain forests, she doesn't expect that Emily will come up with an original piece of work. She knows that Emily will take that information from books and put it on her chart. She might even copy a chart from an encyclopedia, and that's okay.

Following the reasoning of why it is acceptable in this culture for young students to use information for such research, my friend asked me to consider the years and years of thought and knowledge accumulated in Eastern cultures:

> Could it be perhaps, that like our youngest students, teachers in these cultures expect that all thought is, of course, from another source and therefore there is no reason to say that it is? As a matter of fact,

considering the wisdom of the ages, a high school student might seem presumptuous to say that her paper is original.

I would like to do some research on this theory, but true or not, we still need real patience to teach these students the American system of giving credit to others for their ideas. Whatever the risks and whatever the problems, there is no question that our international populations enrich our institutions. At graduation we are accustomed to seeing the quiet, sad goodbyes of young people who have come to mean a great deal to each other. When I observe these exchanges between the international girls, who were once timid and tongue-tied, and the girls from America, I am especially moved. If not for a small New England boarding school, this exchange of learning and, more importantly, of love and understanding could never have happened. These young people bring as much to share with us as we have to share with them. We need to be ready to make time for this exchange within our school communities. Whether we enjoy international dinners, an artists' showcase, homestays, holiday celebrations, or heated ideological exchanges, we have a chance to expose young people to the worthiness of ideas and values which are different from those familiar to them. As our world becomes smaller, and the survival of it depends on how we as a global society can understand and compromise or accommodate, the early friendships of these young people in small schools across our country could someday make a difference in the decisions that will ensure the future of generations.

20

Creating Healthy Communities

by Carol W. Hotchkiss
Director of Counseling Services
Cate School
Carpinteria, California

No matter what we teach, what our catalogues and handbooks espouse or how learned our faculties, it is how we live together in boarding schools that will most affect the character and education of our students. To paraphrase an old saying, "Most students will hear what we say; some students will do what we say; but all students will learn what we do." Our interactions with students and with each other, in and outside the classroom, create a residential community of learning. This concept of community, at times exhausting and intrusive, at other times bonding and rejuvenating, is what defines the special pitfalls and possibilities of a boarding school.

When a new student or faculty member joins a boarding school community, there is no way to adequately prepare her or him for how all-encompassing this new group will become. Work, play, love, friendship, values, music, expressions, dress, success, failure, inclusion, exclusion, meals and sleep are all embodied and influenced by a single, interconnected group of people. Students do not go home from school and faculty do not go home from work. Your teacher is your coach is your dormmaster is your disciplinarian is your confidant. Students become an integral part of a teacher's life and family. The continuity and depth of these relationships create the lasting friendships, memories and camaraderie of even the rockiest boarding school experience. But without the balance of home and school, without the separation of work and personal life, it is critical that boarding schools be attentive to the group dynamics and values of their communities.

All groups, whether a class, a school, a company or a nation, operate simultaneously on two levels. The TASK level is the more understandable and approachable. The TASK is the job to be done, our reason for coming together as a group. School statements of purpose usually define that task. Curriculum, policies, and programs all collaborate to accomplish these goals, our concept of education. If the TASK was all we needed to attend to, our job would be challenging, but relatively straightforward and rational. Teachers could present class material without disruption. Faculty meetings would function logically and efficiently. Students would not be distracted or resistant to the precess of getting a good education.

Groups also function on a more primal, less rational MAINTENANCE level. This is the level of relationships and personal involvement within a group. What are the rules, norms and expectations of this group? What is my role? How can I expect to be treated? For the impatient pragmatist in each of us, this can seem to be an exasperating, irrelevant component of groups. *Unless members feel safe, valued and clear about a group's goals and expectations, however, the group will never efficiently accomplish its task.* We have all sat through faculty meetings during which an apparently simple task (deciding if boys need to wear socks to formal dinner, for instance) becomes a raging battle of controversy and polarization. Sweeping generalizations, personal attacks and disconnected tangents are volleyed about—often with no decision ever being reached. Unless the task is really much more complex than it would appear, it is likely that the MAINTENANCE dynamics of the group are out of whack. I recall an end of year faculty meeting at one school at which I worked. It had been a particularly exhausting, frustrating year and many of the faculty felt unappreciated and ineffective. We summarily expelled 18 troublesome and quite surprised students. These students became a symbol of our growing frustration with the lack of student commitment to the school rules and community. We all have students who enter our classrooms determined to resist, hide or fail no matter what we do or say. Few of us can compete with the personal distractions of the bullied outsider, the lovesick teenager, the drugged-out student or the over-stressed super-achiever. These are all manifestations of MAINTENANCE level concerns that effectively sabotage our efforts to accomplish the task at hand.

Healthy students come from healthy schools. Most students *and* most faculty are shaped, and either strengthened or undermined, by the quality of community life in our schools. Each school is different, but there are, at least, six crucial dynamics that we share when we are healthy and functioning effectively.

Students, faculty, administrators, trustees and parents share a common goal or set of objectives for the community

Each subgroup may have its own personal agenda, but for the school to work as a whole, *there must be a unifying purpose that supersedes individual interests.* We asked our junior class to come up with a list of their objectives—what they wanted to get out of their education. The formation of long-term friendships was high on their list and noticeably absent, as a school objective, from the faculty list. Both groups, however, did share the goals of developing a love of learning and critical thinking, developing an awareness and respect for diversity—and getting into a good college. When we are focused on these goals, the school tends to run smoothly. When our common goals conflict with our divergent interests—completing an assignment versus comforting a friend, for instance—our unity and agreement may break down.

Without a common goal and cooperative effort, the faculty becomes territorial and divisive; students become resistant and combative. Trustees are necessarily concerned about the financial viability of the school, but they must also be committed to making business decisions within the guidelines of the school's educational philosophy and purpose. A common goal allows each participant, adult and adolescent, to share responsibility for school rules, achievement and character. Faculty and administrators support each other's efforts and expertise. Students are actively responsible for their own learning and behavior.

There are healthy adult relationships and role modeling within the community

Students are perceptive and observant of the adults and the adult relationships around them. Their imitations of faculty mannerisms are usually uncanny, and they invariably know faculty gossip long before I do. Since we have a prescribed amount of power in a school community, it is to a student's benefit to understand our quirks, values and vulnerabilities. They have many uninterrupted opportunities to watch us as we teach their classes, coach their teams, manage their dormitories or mingle with our colleagues and families. Temporarily cut off from parents and other adults, students observe us as the adult role models that suggest and define appropriate adult behavior. We are human and imperfect, but a healthy school will support the adults in its community to be the best that we can be. We cannot decry student hazing and sabotage each other or openly humiliate students in our classes. We cannot profess to educate the "whole" student and sacrifice significant aspects of our own personal and family lives. When I had two young children and was running a particularly demanding dormitory, I finally put up a sign on my door that read, "From 5-8 pm is my family time. Unless the dorm is on fire, please wait until 8 to knock." Emergencies, and a few questionable emergencies, did get through, but I was impressed by the number of students who were noticeably moved that I valued and made time for my family.

As adults in a school community, our group dynamics must be healthy and supportive of each other. When faculty members are competitive and cynical with each other, this quickly becomes an acceptable standard for relationships within the community. We must act in accordance with our personal and school values. This is not only an individual obligation, but one which must be supported, protected and valued by the administration and policies of the school.

Faculty should be hired, guided and entrusted to act as ethical role models. Faculty must also have the time and encouragement to develop healthy and satisfying interests beyond their involvement with students. Teaching can be very rewarding, but when we have few other sources of fulfillment, we quickly lose balance and perspective.

There are appropriate roles and expectations which are clear to all community members

Students often don't like or even agree with school rules, but they do like to know where they stand. It is important that students and faculty know what the community limits and expectations are and have a reasonable idea of what will happen if they are violated. Consequences need to be fair and enforceable. A first offense expulsion rule, for instance, gives a strong message about a community rule or value. If it is difficult, even unfair, to enforce in individual situations, however, we either act inconsistently or violate a higher sense of community trust.

Students need adults to be adults with carefully determined values and expectations. Some expectations may be negotiable, most should be reasonable, and all of them must be consistent with our commonly agreed upon objectives. We *are* **us**, and they *are* **them**. This does not have to be a combative relationship, but the lines of distinction between faculty and students should be clear. The intimacy of our residential lives together can make this complicated for both faculty and students. It is impossible and unhealthy for any of us to stay in our teacher/student roles 24 hours a day. When a teacher becomes a buddy, however, students often feel confused or betrayed when he or she must act in a more adult or disciplinarian role. Boarding schools must carefully clarify the varieties and limits of appropriate adult roles.

Teenagers should also be allowed to be teenagers. This means they will make mistakes and question our authority but they must be respected and challenged to learn and grow. In the endless cycle from freshman to senior, we may become callous and wonder when these kids are ever going to grow up. Individually, of course, they do, but our school community remains terminally adolescent. As adults, it is easy to grow impatient with 14-year-old immaturities or 17-year-old rebellions. It is tempting to expect even our youngest students to act more adult. We can forget how scary and lonely it can be to be 14 and living away from home or how difficult it is as a senior leader to supervise and discipline one's peers.

Our demands on students should be realistic, but that does not mean easy or painless. Student responsibilities need to be real and necessary to the school—busy work only undermines a sense of value and responsibility. Students should be encouraged to stretch and allowed to fail. Our impulse to rescue student efforts or "do it better" ourselves, not only robs students of important learning, but also adds more work to our already hectic schedules. When students are trusted and expected to contribute in important and responsible ways, we all begin to work more effectively as a unified community.

There must be a healthy balance of work, play and love for all members of the community

Time is a universal frustration in boarding schools. Students and faculty complain that there is no time to relax, to reflect or to give an adequate amount of attention to their personal relationships. To maintain proper supervision, class and sports offerings and a desired level of individual attention, faculty are often forced into workaholic schedules that are both exhausting and alienating. An overload of academic work, extracurricular activities and student leadership often lead students to the weekend party scene in which, here too, everything is done to excess. Very real demands often make it difficult to choose to give ourselves time for the play and love we need. A headmaster's "free day" inevitably screws up someone's lesson plan. Even some 14 year old students worry about how a spontaneous all-school outing might interfere with their carefully laid plans to get into Harvard. If we don't have fun together, however, we will not work well together. If we don't take time for our friendships and personal reflection, we may get smarter, but we won't get wiser.

Breaking the routine with special activities, speakers or trips gives us time off from the TASK to strengthen and heal the MAINTENANCE level of our school. In January when my dormitory is the sickest, grumpiest, messiest and most unpleasant, I know it is time for a night off of "crazy Olympics" complete with silly contests, singing and lots of food. The lost study time is more than compensated for by our subsequent return to sanity and civilized behavior. Community service, school rituals, twilight leagues and midnight trips to Rocky Horror Picture Show bring a sense of camaraderie and fun that strengthens the whole community. Faculty retreats, skits, antics and activities renew faculty energy and commitment. Healthy schools value and find time for laughter, playfulness and caring within their community.

Healthy schools tolerate differences and respect each individual as an important and valuable member

Everyone belongs. Cruelty, scapegoating, harassment and chronic put downs by students or faculty are not tolerated. That does not mean that everyone likes everyone else or that there is no conflict of ideas or personalities. Conflict is an inevitable and valuable part of groups, relationships and learning. All fully functioning groups must learn to acknowledge conflict and resolve it in such a way that all voices are heard and respected. Class unity and hierarchies are a natural function of maturation and longevity. This ranking, however, should never be allowed to humiliate or degrade anyone. Senior hazing, like child abuse, perpetuates itself—most seniors treat underclass men and women the way they were treated. It is up to schools and carefully observant adults to break any negative cycles. Peer counseling and student leadership programs can help redefine the context of senior power and privilege.

As teachers, we must respect the value and potential of each student with whom we work. It is our job, our profession, to nurture and challenge each individual. One of the most inspiring groups of teachers I ever worked with was in a reform school. The faculty knew their students had problems, many of which were extremely difficult and unpleasant to deal with. Undaunted, the faculty viewed each student as a challenge, an undiscovered gold mine. They shared strategies, celebrated successes, joked good-naturedly and commiserated with each other's frustrations. In our more elite establishments, we sometimes view our students' failings or conflicts as contrived annoyances, rather than the content and challenge of our work. We must remember to focus on the successes on which we can build and the unique strengths and qualities each student brings to our school.

We can only consistently do this if we feel respected and valued. The faculty at the reform school worked as a team sharing ideas, nurturing each other, laughing and, on occasion, crying together. They also had a principal who genuinely appreciated and respected their efforts. He listened, tried to get them what they needed, paid attention to what they were doing and acknowledged both their successes and frustrations. I was a young, slightly shell-shocked teacher, and will never forget my first pay day. Personally amazed that I had survived the first two weeks, I was confronted by the head of the school himself, handing out the paychecks and cold sodas with the hearty congratulations of a coach who knows he has a winning team, no matter what the current score.

Respect filters through a school community. It is learned, or not learned, by the way the faculty treats students—not just the superstar, but the smallest, most difficult student. It is learned, or not learned, by the way the faculty is treated and treats each other. It is learned, or not learned, by how the staff is acknowledged and treated by the entire community. It is learned, or not learned, by who is valued and included in our curriculum, student body, faculty and administration. In healthy schools, each individual is valued for his or her presence, potential and unique contribution to the community.

A healthy school community articulates and lives by consensual values

Healthy boarding schools are ethical communities. We are small, isolated and privileged in many ways that allow us to consciously control our social and moral environment. We can create an enclave of honesty, fairness, kindness and interpersonal responsibility. This is not a common notion in our students' lives today, but it is, nonetheless, essential. We must ask the hard questions and establish a model for ethical behavior. Many of our students just need to have the possibility framed for them. A young, very bright and temporarily confused student who I had been counseling, got herself into some quite serious ethical trouble which would clearly result in her expulsion. She stopped by my house, with her bags packed, ready to run away from both the school and her parents. She was desperately weighing her options for the least painful conclusion to the entire, regrettable mess. After listening to her plans and fears, I asked her,

"What is the *right* thing to do—the choice that will make *you* feel proud of the way you have handled things?" The question visibly surprised her. She thought quietly for a moment, then stood up and said, "I need to go talk to the headmaster."

As ethical communities, we must examine and articulate a common set of values that asks us each to do the right thing. This is not easily or even frequently realized, but stands out as one of the eminent possibilities of a boarding community. One of the times when I believe we most closely realize this potential is during a yearly junior retreat. Focused on a common student/faculty concern about the use of drugs and alcohol in our lives, we quickly reach beyond our differences to the more human questions and personal issues. The only rules for the retreat are confidentiality, no drugs and quiet after 10 p.m. Everything else is run on values—respect for the facilities and for each other, honesty, trust, empathy, personal responsibility and kindness. Dr. Robert Gilkeson, a researcher and speaker on marijuana, attended this retreat in 1986. He was moved and impressed by the "unselfconscious kindnesses . . . the good sportsmanship and fun . . . and the honesty, interest and courtesy" shown by students and faculty during his stay. He went on to note:

> Nothing can duplicate the opportunity of a 24 hour school. . . . It is in these types of institutions that we can still develop students with the feelings and ability to identify with other people, to recognize what is really valuable and important in the world. . . . These students may grow into the sort of adults that have some chance of changing things. . . . Only in such a setting can we construct the environment and the way the people in it deal with each other, providing viable proof that real and pragmatic communities *can* exist and operate successfully within a value system that others like to insist can only exist in an 'ideal,' but 'unreal' society.

As towers of educational privilege, boarding schools are not exempt from the loneliness, meanness, insurrections or temptations of any other school or group. We have unique pressures of supervision, blended roles and an uninterrupted peer culture both for students and adults. We also have the size and constraints to harness what is best in each of us. By creating a healthy school community, we unleash our own potential to teach and our students' potential to grow into healthy responsible adults.

21

A Young
Faculty Perspective

by Kristin Duethorn
Hyde School
Bath, Maine

The thought of being a dorm parent at age 22 scared me because I could not see myself as that type of together person who possessed an unlimited source of advice. I was also unsure of the transition between the freedom of college and the fish bowl existence of living in the dorm. I knew from my own experiences at boarding school that dorm parents unconsciously affect and influence students; this also frightened me. I was constantly afraid of making mistakes or being in situations in which I had no idea what to do. I was sure that the students would not respect me, so I tried hard to make myself appear older in both my looks and actions. I was afraid of the parents who had difficulty separating me from the students, and I could not believe they trusted me; I was sure they questioned my lack of experience. I did.

During these first two years working at a boarding school, I have learned that it is necessary to forget many of the images associated with being a professional. Doing so required a risk I was unwilling to take my first year at Hyde. I hid behind the safety net which traditional images provided. I dressed in clothing that represented the world of professionalism. I tried my best to appear experienced and show the students that if you work hard enough, you can get whatever you want. I learned to give the safe answers to questions and to eliminate any personal associations from the responses. I could give the appropriate response to a possibly precarious question about sex, but I did not dare give a response which reflected my own beliefs, or more importantly, the best interest of the student. When I discovered that the stiff, perfectionist role was not working, I moved to the other extreme. Since I had seen my own dorm parents as friends when I was in school, I spent the rest of my first year trying desperately to be friends with my students. I thought that this would make them like me and would help avoid confrontations. I even believed it would make them want to perform better in the classroom. If they liked me, would they not behave? However, I learned painfully that kids want to be inspired, and that inspiration could come from them seeing me for who I am. I finished the year feeling unfulfilled because I saw no reflection of myself or who I was in the school, and I began to question my choice of careers.

I chose teaching because I felt there was so much I could bring to students. I hoped it was different and wanted it to be exciting. I did not realize that the teachers whom I admired, who had allowed me to enter into their lives, had done so by risking a part of themselves. That first year I sacrificed my values and ignored my conscience while drawing a dishonest picture of who I was. I realize how much of my first year was controlled by my own fears. I had tried to cover them and make them disappear; but I had to confront them if I was to become the role model and influence I wished to be. I do not think that many kids disliked me that first year—that was the safety behind the image—but I also knew that not many kids respected me.

It is now, at the end of my second year at Hyde, that I realize the important role honesty plays in student and faculty relationships. As a young and new faculty member, I had difficulty acting on my conscience. I allowed my insecurities to rule my decisions and I justified them with statements like: "I am sure the students know more about this than I do." This was especially true, for example, when I saw a senior acting inappropriately during study hall. The seniors are given many responsibilities and freedoms. We do not have a student handbook, but live by five words and five principles. As a result, most confrontations are a reaction of conscience and not some fear or need to enforce a rule. To confront a senior or any student would require me to expose and defend my conscience. It would be easier to simply point to a rule. Confronting a senior who has independent study becomes a matter of choice. Many times during my first year, I would walk by without saying a word. There was no rule and therefore I felt myself under no obligation. Maybe I was wrong about the situation, and the student knew better than I. Or, even worse, maybe nobody on the faculty would back me up. Nonetheless I still thought what he was doing was wrong. Even when I had the courage to say something, I felt vulnerable because there was no rule to support me. When the seniors challenged me, I most often retreated. It took me that first year to understand how truth, conscience and concern, three of the school's words or principles, connected. Those seniors were not pursuing activities which lead to their best work. I had to show concern for them while simultaneously respecting my conscience. As time went on, I realized that students trusted faculty members who acted on conscience and were not afraid to speak their minds. Ironically, the same students who challenged me, told me at faculty evaluations that I needed to have more confidence and stand up for myself.

I struggled similarly in the classroom. I tried imitating other teachers and their styles. I lost my own personality in the classroom but loved the security that came from "success." I had relatively few discipline problems and we were covering the material. I found it difficult to learn from other teachers and, at the same time, be myself. So many of my own ideas and thoughts about teaching were pushed back into my head. I began to enjoy being in the classroom less because those ideas contained the excitement I had wanted to bring into my classroom. Finally, another faculty member told me to share my struggle with my classes. I felt extremely uncomfortable and worried that, by admitting my weaknesses, I would never regain the control over the classroom. Surprisingly, the students helped me to see that this same control which I valued was keeping us from reaching our potential as a class. We needed to struggle and experience difficulty. We needed to see how we reacted to stress and excitement. By playing it safe, I was keeping the class from learning and protecting everyone from the truth. I was too afraid to see who they were and to risk sharing who I was. After sharing my problem, the atmosphere in the classroom changed. More ideas and feelings were expressed because of a trust that had developed. I did not like the pit I felt in my stomach for the first few weeks, but it made me feel awake and forced me to learn. I know that my own teachers were not as in control as they made themselves appear, but I also know that few took the risk of sharing their fears with their students. This new freedom in the classroom allowed me to speak my conscience more often and to push the limits of the class without the fear of being unsuccessful.

The time around 9:30 p.m. when study hall is over and the knocking begins at my door has become my favorite part of the day. The conversation with the students is more stimulating and important especially when we both can let down the images we try so hard to portray during the day. I realize that it is in these situations that teaching truly occurs and that honesty is essential. Students feel free enough to come down and discuss the issues confronting their lives. I feel that too often dorm parents imitate the relationships many kids have with their parents where honest communication is avoided. Parents want to preserve the harmony of the family and are afraid of what their kids are doing. As a dorm parent, I see it as my job to create an atmosphere in which kids know they can talk about anything without the fear of disapproval or discipline. I also feel that, because I am a young faculty member, the students feel more comfortable talking to me. I feel good and know the relationship is honest when students call me during their vacations to share successes and struggles; I know our relationship has moved beyond the structure of daily school life.

Normally topics include: academics, drugs, family life, friends, parents, sex, and self-esteem. My first year, I avoided these conversations or tried to close them as quickly and easily as possible. I had made the mistake of believing that being a dorm parent implied perfection. I had picked up some common phrases of advice and distributed them generically like aspirin to soothe all pain. Again,

I did now want to be caught without the answer or say something the school would feel was inappropriate. Students need to hear the truth which has been avoided many times by their own parents. Frequently students want to talk about sex and relationships or drugs. I used to feel uncomfortable sharing my own experience on any of these subjects. I have discovered, however, that the kids learn the most when I share with them, and an automatic trust develops. Moreover, many of the issues they struggle with are still fresh in my mind. Nobody here at Hyde has tried to regulate how much or how little I say. I feel comfortable sharing my most personal experiences when I feel it will benefit the student.

During the past two years, it has become easier to share my own experience with students. The week before a parents' weekend always seems intense and full of emotion. Typically a student will come to my apartment confused and needing help to sort out mixed emotions. Recently, one student, whose parents have been divorced for years, was afraid of seeing her father for the first time in three years. I helped her work through her feeling of love, anger, loss and fear. I validated many of her feelings through my similar experience of having divorced parents and shared the mistakes I had made in dealing with the same issue. I warned her that she could not use her feelings as an excuse for her behavior over the weekend. Her struggle brought back vivid memories for me, and I knew I understood what she was feeling. When her father arrived that weekend, I watched from my apartment as they greeted each other after the long separation. As I watched the tears run down her face, I felt the moisture on my own. An unbelievable connection to this student formed immediately. Two minutes later, she knocked on my door because she wanted me to meet her father. At that moment, I shared with her what was going on with me and why I felt so emotional. I shared my own feelings of inadequacy and realized that there was still a part of my own past that needed to be resolved. Our bond has been special since that day. Not all moments in the dorm are going to be this dramatic, but there is always the potential as long as we are open to sharing on an honest level.

Another busy week is the time before a vacation. It is during these times that students begin to worry about the standards they are going to set for themselves over the break. They need to talk about their sexual behavior, their relationship with parents, and the role that drugs and alcohol play in their lives. It is part of our role as dorm parents and educators to be concerned with how our students conduct themselves over breaks. I do not remember any discussions on this topic when I was at boarding school. I feel fortunate to work at a school that deals with truth and not image. This atmosphere can only contribute to the quality of residential life. The environment is less motivated by fear, and the students have the opportunity to deal with their issues without being judged or thrown out of school. The students do not feel afraid to speak honestly about how they have spent their vacations. Many students today truly want help, but are too afraid to risk the consequences of telling the truth. Part of this fear stems from the fact that most of the adults in their lives have not shared their own weaknesses. It is important then that students see faculty struggle with their own lives and understand that hitting an obstacle is not a sign of failure and that much of your character depends on how you deal with the issue. It is sometimes difficult to have an open relationship with a student because you can learn things you do not want to know. I have had many conversations with students on how they were going to spend their breaks. A couple of students have said they would give up smoking but not drinking. As a faculty member, I need to encourage them not to drink and to remind them it is illegal. I also, however, have a respect for the individual students and their commitment to honesty. I do not need to pressure them with an image of perfection. I can accept them for who they are and help them move forward. The students respect this approach and are not afraid to come and talk with faculty.

In order to have this type of relationship with students, they must learn how to control their own lives. Hyde places responsibility on the individual to act according to conscience and not out of fear of a student handbook, whose lessons do not move beyond the gates of a school. Hyde bases its philosophy on five words (courage, concern, curiosity, integrity, and leadership) and five principles (truth, conscience, destiny, humility and Brother's Keeper) in order to teach character; this is the primary focus of the school. Each student hopefully learns to internalize these words. Moreover, the senior's graduation status is based on the standards by which they have chosen to live their lives. Merely completing academic credits does not insure a Hyde School diploma. The seniors and faculty spend over forty hours together during the last semester of school talking about what they have learned and how they plan to apply it to their lives. Through this process the words and principles, unlike a student handbook, follow the student beyond the gates of Hyde.

When I came to Hyde School, I was surprised with the level of responsibility that was given to the students. A residential program needs to allow students the opportunity to practice making decisions in their lives; it cannot protect the students by controlling their lives and keeping them safe. Every student has a facilities job (dishwasher, classroom cleaner) and a dorm job. Both of these areas are supervised completely by students. The students also run the Dean's Area of the school where they must get involved in other students' lives. In the Dean's Area students discuss, implement and supervise school discipline. The seniors in all of these areas work closely creating a unique bond. Thus the senior class determines the tone of the school. They struggle with their leadership position and learn how to work together. This responsibility leads to a sense of pride in and commitment to the school. My dorm runs by similar guidelines. Students (seniors for the majority of the year) check rooms at night, do lights out, conduct room inspection, and run study hall and the jobs program. They also devise and enforce the majority of the dorm policies. They confront one another on their actions and deal responsibly with supervising discipline. I like the way in which this process gives me the opportunity to be a resource and friend as opposed to an enforcer of rules. Because of this relationship, the dorm is more of a home and less a part of an institution for both faculty and students. I have even gone into the dorm looking for answers to my own problems. The kids understand that we as faculty are not perfect and have problems too. This mutual understanding leads to a quality of respect I do not remember having in my own school.

This respect leads to a unity among all areas of the school. We meet as a whole school once a week to discuss any current issues in the school. The students are allowed to voice their own opinions and their ideas often influence life within the community. Ultimately, I feel that the bond between all students and faculty is strong because we have seen both the strengths and weaknesses in each other and have tried to live in an environment of honest friendship. Often the atmosphere is uncomfortable and changing. I believe this provides the opportunity for maximum growth as individuals which less intense, more comfortable environments do not encourage. This acceptance of one another, and the idea that we must all continually develop ourselves, allows both faculty and students to let go of protective images.

I have found it very difficult to live in an environment based on truth, although it is less stressful than being forced to hide behind an image. It has taught me to take a good look at myself and how I lead my life. All faculty at residential schools need to be involved in a continuous learning process and persevere through success and failure. The students must see how faculty deal with their lives; it is through this that the students learn. I feel that I am truly a teacher when the majority of my teaching occurs outside of the classroom. By committing myself to this process of truth, I have naturally gained the respect I was so worried about achieving at the beginning of my career.

22

Tightening up the Residential Program: Dorm Faculty Accountability

by Ed Stansfield, Director of Admission
Kimball Union Academy
Meriden, New Hampshire

Four years ago, after six years as a full-time English teacher, dorm master and coach at Kimball Union, I assumed the post of director of admission. The most striking aspect of this move has been, primarily, my direct, bottom-line accountability to the headmaster. I still live in a dorm, but find direct accountability in this realm, beyond that which I personally feel, to be nearly absent except in the occasional crisis situation. My premise is that many boarding schools unfortunately take a laissez faire approach to their residential programs. After nine years in dormitories, I have come to firmly believe that there is a significant curriculum at work in boarding school residential programs. Not a new idea. I intend to suggest how the current dorm faculty structure at most boarding schools can be used to significantly improve the effectiveness of the residential program—improvements founded in greater dorm faculty accountability. While all school administrators worry about the increased time commitment this may cause—possibly stealing from class preparation—no school can afford to ignore the societal and demographic changes that make it necessary for a residential program to focus on student needs which in the past have been satisfied at home. The residential curriculum, like the mathematics or English curriculum, requires constant attention and maintenance to ensure that what students learn in the dormitory is consistent with the mission and direction of the school. To accomplish this task and therefore make a residential program successful, schools must develop a level of administration among dorm heads.

I do not intend to compare or impose my experience with administrative accountability upon dorm faculty, although administration of a school and administration of a dorm are quite similar. Dorm faculty, however, administer and advance their curriculum in often intangible and certainly unquantifiable territory. It is, therefore, important that on-site management be present and active. Schools must encourage and train dorm heads to act as managers of those who work and live in their dorms. Dorm staff must be willing to speak with student residents about a myriad of issues from personal to academic and social. Dormitory heads must do the same with dorm faculty as well as with students. Faculty are often made dorm heads after accumulated years of experience in dorm living; however, neither expertise as a teacher, experience in a dorm, nor just "being good with kids" means that a faculty member will necessarily be a suitable manager of a dormitory.

Most agree, in principle, with what I have just stated, but in many schools the practical side of dorm management, which ultimately means person-to-person accountability, is left to a central authority, such as the headmaster, assistant headmaster or dean. This tendency to leave student and/or dormitory staff accountability to an absentee administrator is akin to reading Yeats with an English class and never providing any historical gloss nor discussing the work. Some students will pick up hints of the meaning but will have no framework in which to understand the piece or reach a conclusive meaning. Other students will go off on a wild interpretive venture and somehow manage to free-associate an erroneous meaning. No responsible teacher of English would practice this. My point is that someone must be there to encourage and enhance sound understanding. Metaphorically, it is not enough to simply read the verse. Neither is it enough just to have "good people" working and living in the dormitory.

I am not advocating the restructuring of faculty priorities as though our central responsibility were something other than our students' academic achievement. Increased emphasis on residential life, however, will require an increased time commitment. Fortunately the present structures of dorm faculties in most boarding schools are sufficient to make the residence programs more effective without major restructuring, but accountability must be the focus.

Dorm faculty accountability can be achieved in a number of ways including annual evaluation by student residents, annual evaluation by the dormitory head, and most importantly, active, on-site management by the dormitory head. He must hold dorm faculty and student residents accountable. He should focus on creating a management team with the other dormitory faculty and fostering dormitory faculty unity. This can be accomplished through communication on both the formal level of regular dormitory meetings and informal level of daily contact with dormitory faculty. Informal communication is an essential element to on-site faculty management by the dormitory head. The combination will discourage deferring to assumed standards of dormitory expectations. Formal and informal levels of communication reinforce each other and create a foundation for accountability.

Four years ago I headed a dormitory of about 20 boys. I lived in an attached house and a single faculty member lived in an apartment in the dormitory. During that year we shared concern for a student who was acting up and we feared was getting involved in illicit activities. We both had personally spoken to him and compared notes with one another on a number of occasions. The student failed to modify his behavior significantly, and we agreed the situation called for resolution. We separately collected data from dormitory residents, teachers, and coaches for three days. When we met to make a decision, we were disconcerted that based on virtually the same information, we each had formed quite separate ideas of the resolution required. We vigorously discussed our opposing views, felt frustrated, shared our reasoning, understood one another's separate intentions, identified our common goals, and formulated a compatible plan. Before we could express our resolution to the student, we worked out all the specifics on paper: who would speak to the student, what would be said, and what sanctions would be imposed.

This is an example of what I refer to as on-site management by the dorm head. It requires time and is not arrived at easily, but it does build a management team and dorm faculty unity. I believe it is important in large and small dormitories alike to establish this foundation for accountability so that practices don't vary widely and send an inconsistent message to students within the dorm.

Varying levels and degrees of faculty and, thus, student accountability can cause wide variations in dormitory management. The worst pits what students see as "good" faculty against "bad." Dormitory reputations form along these lines. I concede that variations between dormitories will forever exist due to the nature of faculty personalities involved, but I suggest that too wide a variation can be divisive. To avoid this, dormitory heads and staff must agree in principle with the goals of the residence program. To do this they must maintain regular contact with each other to ensure that their agreed-upon principle is represented in the practical application of rules and regulations within and among all dormitories.

When our dormitory heads at Kimball Union began to meet on a consistent basis there was wide disagreement and, as you might expect, arguments. The dormitory heads needed almost a full year of regular meetings to identify the common ground on which our residence program presently operates. The process takes time. Lest you be misled, the outcome for our school has not been pandorm harmony nor total faculty agreement. The positive outcome for our school has been the institution of an ongoing process that is constantly establishing, affirming and/or altering the principles and practices that support and advance our school's mission. It is therefore important that the dormitory faculty and dormitory head are together responsible for overseeing the residents and for deriving regular meeting agenda items from their experiences with student residents.

Since a change in administrations three years ago, we have moved from a dean-central system of student accountability to a less central on-site system of student accountability in the dormitories. For instance, under the past administration, if a student threw a water balloon in the dormitory, he or she would have been reported to the dean who would have enforced some type of sanction. The problem with this system was a lack of immediate, consequential feedback for the infraction. The "official" consequence was not delivered until the dean had made a decision which sometimes took days.

Under our current system, dormitory staff are encouraged to deal with minor infractions, such as the water balloon, on the spot and communicate the infraction and sanction to the dormitory head and dean. Sanctions may be along the lines of taking out the dormitory trash for a day or two, cleaning the dorm lounge, or staying in one's room after study hours. The advantage is that the consequences are direct and related. Does this mean that fewer students are tossing around water balloons? Probably not; but it does provide the student with consequences directly related to his or her actions. They learn this in the classroom; why else give the unannounced quiz? Learning the lesson of consequence should be part of the curriculum in the dormitory as well.

Dorm heads should be chosen for and trained in management and information organization skills. We have always done dormitory head training in-house with very little distinction from how we train dormitory faculty. I believe that dormitory head training would benefit from an off-campus management seminar or an on-campus management consultancy workshop. The important difference between dormitory heads and staff is that the head will have to manage adult peers. It is only sensible that the dormitory head be equipped with managerial techniques in motivation, performance evaluation, praise, and non-performance follow-up.

Not every faculty member who is "good in the dorm" possesses the necessary skills to manage peers. The dormitory head must have the skills not only to work and live in a close community with his or her peers but to be able to successfully deal with the added complexities management requires. The dormitory head must be able to approach other dorm faculty on professional issues and individual performance. Since this administrative status will mean an increase in time commitment, just as with academic department heads, the administration must give the dormitory head allowances (for necessary meetings with dorm faculty, performance evaluation of dorm faculty, interviewing job candidates for dorm faculty openings, time alone, and contemplation about whether he or she is doing the right thing).

The potential liability of creating an active administration at the dormitory level is the increased departmentalization of a faculty. Such a schism will be discouraged by the proposed participation of dorm faculty in the school administration. Secondarily, dorm heads may feel isolated and should be encouraged by the school to develop a sense of professionalism and camaraderie among themselves, a process which we have found to be harder than it sounds.

Trying to establish camaraderie between dorm heads is like trying to establish camaraderie between academic department heads: personalities and departmental or dormitory sovereignty get in the way. But while academic department heads tend to have a strong sense of professionalism, this is often altogether absent in dormitory heads. We have found, however, that the increased administrative activity of the dormitory heads and staff can contribute to its development. Our school has encouraged this development by having dorm heads organize on-campus workshops put on by outside consulting groups, spend more time and effort on inter-school training of new faculty dorm residents, and write formal evaluations of dorm faculty.

The school has much to gain by creating a dormitory level of administration: the individual dormitory head takes an active role in the administration of a dormitory rather than a passive role directed by an absentee dean; the school develops and maintains a strong residential component, cultivates important faculty skills and increases the number of faculty/administrators who are invested in the school and its direction; most important, all of these benefits deepen the school's culture by making the dorm heads leaders.

Dorm heads should be accountable to a dean of students (or dean of residence) through monthly meetings and annual evaluations. The same guidelines for communication within the dormitory apply to the relationship between the dean and dormitory head. Again communication builds a foundation for accountability. As a leader, the dorm head should be instrumental in managing the flow of information to and from his or her staff and residents. The dorm head should generate meeting agenda for the dean's meeting, dorm staff meetings, and student proctor meetings. He or she should also be sure to share the meeting agenda from one group with the other two groups and vice versa. The consistent flow of information from one group to the next and back is imperative. This issue is of such importance that it is worth an example: the dorm heads have their regular meeting with the dorm staff at which they will discuss a specific agenda derived from within the dormitory. At the monthly dean's meeting they should present those agenda items that seem most important in their individual dorms. They should take from the dean's meeting the agenda discussed there and share it with the dorm faculty to get their comments and disperse the information shared by the other dorm heads and the dean. In short, this process should work in the same manner in which most academic departments work. The origin of agenda items should be at the dormitory level. Consequently, dormitory meetings need to be organized around agendas and not just be opportunities for dorm staff to get together and discuss the latest crisis.

I realize that this is a level of organization and managerial responsibility with which many dorm heads and staff are unfamiliar and uncomfortable. It is no wonder; the demands that such a system puts on the dorm heads and the possible stress it can place on the relationship with other dorm faculty can make dorm living more complex than it already is. But consider the benefits: the potential elimination of the regrettably common faculty experience of listening each September to the head's or dean's decrees of how they have improved the residence program over the summer to ensure its success this year. This annual ritual is emblematic of the current pyramid administrative structure in many (not all) schools. I submit that an active and organized level of dormitory heads and staff (this goes for academic department heads also) can be successful at inverting the pyramid structure and getting the accurate and proper information to trickle down to the person at the top who ultimately must make the decisions which determine the direction of the school.

Conclusion
"Great Ideas":
Communication on a
National Level

by Louis M. Crosier

This is the heart of the boarding school promise: that some adult will become involved in the life of each child, will come to care about that child's growth and development, and that caring will make a difference in the child's education.

Bill Poirot & Dusty Richard

Relationship is the heart of the boarding school promise. Despite the extremely different philosophies, structure, style and rules of the schools represented in *Healthy Choices, Healthy Schools*, all the authors agree, as Burch Ford writes, "the most effective learning takes place in the context of a relationship." Relationship transcends rules and is the true motivating factor at boarding schools. Jim Adams writes, "When the relationship is more human than official, its obligations are more moral than legal; and when a student senses a moral obligation, a few implicit expectations will accomplish much more than a raft of explicit rules." Bill Poirot and Dusty Richard incorporate relationship and accountability into a system:

> Children should be encouraged by the school's rooming process to choose adults with whom they have a shared interest or existing relationship. Adults should ask for students in their dorm on the same basis, and when the school gets to the last five kids to be assigned rooms, it will know who is in the most need of connecting with an adult.

Formalized Systems

Once a school decides what values it wants to institutionalize, it should create formal systems to ensure these values are upheld. For example, if a school says it values diversity, this should be reflected in its daily operation. If it values leadership, then it will benefit from a well-designed student prefect program such as the one Susan Graham describes. This includes an application process, a clear set of goals, an action plan, a system of communication, and a process for evaluation and feedback. The generic "regular meetings" are less effective than the clearly defined "dinner meeting every Monday night to discuss the weekend and prepare for the week ahead." Schools should work toward a formal system for every aspect of school life which they value—hiring, training, evaluation, and so on. It is an ongoing process, of course, but the commitment to build a system, such as Loomis Chaffee's anti-drug, anti-alcohol program demonstrates an understanding of what it takes to create the foundation for a healthy residential community.

How about a handbook which describes each system? "A Dormitory Staff Handbook is a must," writes Susan Graham. Jim Wilson describes his experience: "We put together a handbook for faculty on how to respond to a whole series of situations—from slight suspicion (a student simply acting strangely at a dorm check-in for example) to the situation in which a faculty member walks into a room where a joint is being shared or a beer is being drunk." Is it overkill to have so many handbooks? I don't think so. I certainly would have benefitted from clear guidelines on specific systems. These handbooks should be shared between schools. Among all the NAIS schools, there should already be an impressive collection of handbooks, most of which probably grew out of specific crises. Together these might help your school take a pro-active stance on several of the challenges which lie ahead in the next academic year.

The Three "A"s of Positive Change

Awareness

The voices in *Healthy Choices, Healthy Schools* suggest that schools must fine tune their awareness of the importance and intricacies of the residential side of a 24-hour community. Poirot and Richard write: "I am suggesting that even in most boarding schools, the issue of dormitory life is not central to the school's self-image. The faculty in most boarding schools are divided on the subject and I am afraid that, even among the dormitory parents, only a few see their work as absolutely central to the worth of the school." Mark Timmerman shows that sleeping and eating, for example, affect students' lives more deeply than we might have previously acknowledged. Certainly the structure of many residential programs does not reflect adequate concern for these issues. Michael Williamson, Jan Gilley, Pamela Brown, and Torrence Burrowes underscore the importance of looking more closely at how we can serve all members of our communities. Dan Heischman suggests we sometimes think we are working in the best interest of the kids but, by neglecting our own needs, we often convey the wrong message. Clearly, an awareness of the systems we have or don't have in place and the message we send students and colleagues is the first step toward creating healthier boarding schools. As a start, I suggest individual schools heighten their awareness of residential issues of specific concern by undertaking a process similar to NAIS's Multicultural Assessment Plan. Schools could create their own Dormitory Assessment Plan which might begin with the kinds of questions Bill Poirot and Dusty Richard pose in their "Dormitory Audit." NAIS might well serve member schools by developing a service along these lines.

Attitude

The next step in creating healthier schools is to develop and nurture a problem-solving attitude among students and faculty, a belief that constructive change is possible and desirable. Although it is not easy to continuously look for the good side of situations, thinking in terms of solutions is essential. In the short run it is easier to avoid confronting issues of concern but ultimately this drains the community because the problem becomes ingrained and institutionalized. To develop healthy systems like Loomis Chaffee's anti-drug, anti-alcohol program, community members need to commit to being part of the solution rather than part of the problem. Schools should create formats for addressing problems. For example, when a faculty member or student identifies a problem, or has a complaint, he should be sure to voice it loud and clear but accompany it with three possible solutions and the impact these might have on the community.

The most beneficial attitude for problem solving is one that embraces diversity. Openness to perspectives other than one's own allows new ideas to enter a community and creative solutions to surface. An attitude which may seem as specific as accepting racial, cultural or gender differences has broad sweeping implications for how we approach our work with colleagues and students. As Joy Sawyer Mulligan notes, a "Why on earth?" attitude has no place in a community interested in self-improvement. Michael Williamson shares a similar perspective, highlighting the inappropriateness of the statement "I can't relate." Jan Gilley writes: "It is essential that we build not just tolerance for other beliefs and customs, but interest in them and respect for them." This attitude should apply not only to international students and students of color, but to all members of the community. The process of self-examination which grows out of a commitment to diversity can be an uncomfortable one, but a necessary one if we are to improve our effectiveness as teachers. Sarah Jordan writes:

> A primary challenge for the dorm parent is to be sensitive to gender differences and the issues that arise from these. Whether we are "parenting" students of the same sex or of the opposite sex, this should mean examining our own stereotypes about male and female behavior . . . as teachers we have a commitment to continue our own learning, and this includes, in my view, learning about our own emotional patterns and prejudices.

An attitude which acknowledges that we bring our own experience to the way in which we interpret the world will allow us to incorporate, not reject, the rich variety of perspectives and ideas, different from and often opposed to our own, into solutions which will improve the quality of residential life in our schools. Positive change requires acceptance of diversity.

Accountability

There is a difference between policy and systems which actualize policy. Too often policy translates to lip service, or at best inconsistent application. Accountability is the essential ingredient in all systems within a school. Whether it comes in the form of Hyde School's "Brother's Keeper"; John Conner's recommendation that heads and deans circulate visibly in the dorms throughout the year; new levels of administrators within the residential structure as proposed by Ed Stansfield; or feedback to the admission office on the progress of "risk admits," as suggested by Joy Sawyer Mulligan, accountability is the ingredient which ensures high standards. The ongoing effort to improve residential life stagnates without the element of feedback in every aspect of operation. We have become quite good at holding students accountable, have developed elaborate systems for so doing, and as Burch Ford suggests, they value it: "Kids recognize and respect the courage that it takes to intervene when ignorance, indifference or abdication would be the easier, and perhaps more familiar, position to take." The challenge now is to enhance collegial accountability and support. I believe this begins with bi-weekly two-way evaluations between colleagues. Again Burch Ford suggests, "confrontation is protection, something we all owe others whom we care about."

The Essential Systems

Training

Without exception, every chapter which mentions training of dorm faculty, dorm heads and student prefects calls for more of it. Hamilton Gregg writes, "boarding programs should be pro-active, preparing for every circumstance." He suggests:

> It would make sense to spend money prior to the start of school, teaching new faculty and staff the kind of skills they will need. This would save costs incurred by having to hire a new set of teachers every year. The burn out would be less and the faculty would be more involved and equipped to deal with the complexity of issues they will confront. Without this training they can only cope; they cannot be pro-active and thrive. Most schools finance training sessions too late—after the first year and during the summer months. By then the "wet-behind-the-ears" are beaten, bruised and worn out.

Susan Graham's chapter describes an effective training program for student prefects. It should serve as the model for ongoing faculty training and professional development. Additionally, a formal faculty mentor system can serve as an ongoing source of in-house faculty development. A formal mentoring system within department and within the dorms validates experienced faculty members' expertise while encouraging self-evaluation in a non-threatening way. "You never really learn it until you teach it" in this case applies to mentors. In the same way a teacher learns his subject inside and out by teaching it, the mentor gains a deeper understanding of the qualities of an effective teacher, dorm parent, and administrator by reflecting on the experience and sharing insight with a less experienced teacher. Using the mentoring systems which exist in many academic departments as a model, schools should institute a mentoring system in residential life. Finally, an effective formal mentor program underscores the fact that there are many leaders within the community.

Student prefects

Susan Graham writes: "Acknowledging and training the students who are willing to risk the possibilities and attendant responsibilities of leadership is one of the most important aspects of any residential program." Student leaders provide the all-important bridge between student and adult experience, interpreting and softening the sometimes unwelcome advice of adults and articulating the climate and concerns of the student population. Student leaders play one of the most important roles in any boarding school. Again deferring to Susan Graham: "There is no comparison between life as a dorm director working with trained student leaders and life as a dorm director without." Jim Wilson's description of two junior prefects whose planned intervention on a drug-using sophomore got him the help he needed demonstrates the value of a carefully orchestrated prefect system.

Professional Parenting

"Dorm parent" is a useful title, despite what some schools feel to the contrary. It underscores the importance of kids having parents even if it is only an approximation. However, "dorm parent" should be an earned title, given only to faculty members who by virtue of their experience and age can provide a more realistic approximation of the parenting role. Ed Stansfield proposes professionalizing the residential operating structure by giving dorm heads administrative responsibility. I agree whole-heartedly and would like too hash out his idea a little further. Perhaps, as is the case at many schools, new dorm faculty should begin as "dorm interns." Young faculty should go by a different title ("dorm coach" or "resident advisor") which they earn through a year's formal training and hands-on experience. There would be an additional step before earning the "dorm parent" or dorm head status. This step might be called "dorm associate" and could be earned after young faculty had additional formal training and experience in counseling and began to develop an individual style and rituals (like John Conner's "room inspection sheets" and "word of the day"). The next step, if appropriate, would be into the position of "dorm parent," a role recognized by a significant pay increase and the renaming of the dorm (per Groton School). In addition to normal duty, the "dorm parent" would take on an administrative role, cutting down on classroom work slightly, but keeping the hours in the dorm the same. Moving from one rung to the next should not be automatic, and each school should determine its own criteria for advancing its staff. Titles and clear job descriptions convey a great deal in an environment of minimal pay increases, and they help establish a clear understanding of the differences in expectations at each level of the job. At all levels, from "intern" to "dorm parent," faculty members would be expected to hold students accountable, but the dorm parent would be viewed as someone to whom students could go with significant parenting concerns. Failing to differentiate between levels of expertise by giving all faculty the same title in the dorm suggests that anyone could do the job (i.e. the job is easy or has little importance). Former "dorm parents" or dorm heads who have retired from the dorm and moved into other campus housing could serve as "dorm mentors." This would connect the most experienced faculty with a residence hall, providing the dorm head with another source of advice, validating the expertise of veteran faculty members, and keeping the community a tightly knit whole.

Defining *in loco parentis* poses one of the greatest challenges facing prep schools today. How far should boarding schools go in assuming responsibilities normally held by the family? The question is particularly acute in contemporary society where, as Ed Stansfield suggests, "no school can afford to ignore the societal and demographic changes that make it necessary for a residential program to focus on student needs which in the past have been satisfied at home." Although we cannot take the place of the natural parents we have an obligation to teach our students how to make healthy choices beyond the classroom, which in the words of Kristin Duethorn "are not left behind at the school's gate when the students leave."

Healthy Choices, Healthy Schools is about attitude, relationship, accountability and communication. As a collection, it is only a small sample of the "great ideas" harbored in the collective experience of faculty, administrators and broader constituencies of prep schools across the nation. The importance of communication between colleagues and between schools should not be underestimated. The opportunity for community members to discuss residential issues should be ongoing and facilitated by regional and national organizations like NAIS. I suggest that *Independent School* magazine and others devote a regular column to specific issues of boarding life including lights-out, telephone, shower and parietals rules, formal meals, the weekend program, study hall and compensation. Faculty members from different schools could write about their school's policy, procedures and philosophy. Call it, "How Other Schools Do

It." I find it fascinating and helpful to learn about the differing systems at prep schools because I remember how isolated I felt in my own work in the dorm. For some reason I believed all schools were structured similarly and shared the same problems. Clearly this is not the case. I hope that schools will reach out to each other to share their "great ideas" with increasing frequency.

Did You Borrow This Book? Want a Copy of Your Own?

Need To Learn More About Private Schools And How To Work With Young Adults?

ORDER FORM

YES, I want to increase my knowledge and **RECEIVE A 20% DISCOUNT** by owning Louis Crosier's new book *Healthy Choices, Healthy Schools* and his first book on private schools, *Casualties of Privilege*. Send me _____ sets for the low price of $27.95 per set.

YES, I want to learn more about running a dormitory and managing young adults. Send me _____ copies of Louis Crosier's new book *Healthy Choices, Healthy Schools* at $19.95 per copy.

YES, I want to learn more about the current social issues confronting the private school world today. Send me _____ copies of Louis Crosier's book *Casualties of Privilege* at $14.95 per copy.

Please **add $1.85 per book for shipping and handling.** Canadian or other foreign orders must be accompanied by a postal money order in U.S. Funds. Allow 30 days for delivery. Send check payable to: Avocus Publishing, Inc., 1223 Potomac Street, N.W., Washington, D.C. 20007. Credit card orders may be called in toll free to: (800)345-6665.

Name _____

Phone ( ) _____

Address _____

City/State/Zip _____

Here's my check/money order for $ _____

Bill my: VISA   MasterCard   American Express

   Acc. # _____

   Signature _____

   Expires _____

BULK ORDERS DISCOUNTED

For bulk discount prices please call (202) 333-8190

LEARN HOW YOU CAN BECOME AN AVOCUS AUTHOR

Avocus Publishing, Inc. develops and publishes group-authored books on timely social issues. The goal of the books is to encourage meaningful dialogue and promote healthy, responsible choices. Avocus books focus on educational practice and policy, adolescent health and first amendment rights. Contributing authors include professors and secondary school teachers, family planning professionals, doctors, attorneys, arts administrators and many others. Authors have spoken on national radio and television including: National Public Radio, Christian Science Monitor Radio, and the Phil Donohue Show.

Avocus Publishing, Inc. does not discriminate on the basis of race, color, creed, religion, nationality, gender, or sexual orientation. To learn more about current Avocus projects and to receive a Forthcoming Books list, send a self addressed stamped envelope to Avocus Publishing, Inc., attn. Claire Pyle, Senior Editor, 1223 Potomac Street, N.W., Washington, D.C. 20007.